AIM HIGH PUSH HARD

Ahmed Gbadamosi, Physician Associate

Aim High Push Hard

Copyright © 2023

All Rights Reserved

ISBN: 979-8-218-28484-8

Aim High Push Hard

Dedication

My Professors, My Patients, My Preceptors, My Classmates, who called me obnoxious for asking too many questions, when all I was trying to do was learn medicine from the seams, like a hand-woven fabric, from the inside out, I internalized medicine intrinsically. I wanted to be the best of the best. That's just what I am. Do not mistake confidence for arrogance. Let me shine baby. Future President of The United States of America. This is only the beginning. The road is long.

My Highschool Guidance Counselor, for seeing something in me that I didn't see in myself. "An Academic Giant," I had behavioral issues, my environment taught me how to feel that way. I had to learn to become violent 'cause the wolves in my section were violent, in order to survive my neighborhood, otherwise the predators would've preyed on me and I would not have survived the jungle to write this novel today. But you scrutinized my GPA and realized something didn't add up. You said, "The guys you hang around all have 'F's," on their report card and criminal record, You're a straight "A" student."

Thank you for asking me to take the SAT's and apply to college, if it wasn't for you. Who knows where the trajectory of my life would've gone? I was infatuated with street-life. By 11th grade I was neck deep in hustling, making more money than my teachers. But I knew there was an end, it was only a matter of time. However, the only way that I was going to leave was on a stretcher, or in a pine box. 25yrs in a jail cell? Buried alive? SheeeedN'me, I'd rather die. You changed the course of my life. I'm grateful to have met you.

Aim High Push Hard

Dr. Allen Tustin, thank you for not giving in. Always exhorting me to check my sources before I do my research on infectious diseases and never allowing me to ask you a question unless I meticulously analyzed the question and answered it myself first, no matter how ambiguous the answer was to me, because you weren't going to give me an answer. You wanted me to become familiar with "figuring medicine out for yourself." You were the most challenging professor I ever had in my entire life, and you came to class every day on a peritoneal dialysis machine. I can't imagine how excruciating that was for you. I appreciate you.

You didn't teach for money, you taught for the love of medicine. Many students fled the classroom because you were adamant about medicine being arduous. You either have what it takes, or you don't. You were the epitome of "Where does the want meet the need and the need meets the want?"

Aim High Push Hard

Medicine isn't for everybody. Give me my "nickels" I diagnosed a couple zebras Dr. Tustin. But you were right! I diagnosed plenty more horses than zebras. You're the reason I listen for hooves when patients come in.

Gregory Horne, aka "Quack" Rock Creek, Hot Boy: You taught me to always feel as good as I look and look as good as I feel. The honey-hole that we are all ascending to reach, knowing we will never get there. You taught me to be fearless bruh'. When everyone chastised me 'cause I didn't want to leave school early to chase that paper. You told me, "Go for whachu' know bruh', the hood ain't going nowhere."

Tyrone Hopkins, aka "Say $tik'em next time." You taught me about life and work. Instead of coming in set, sturdy, locked in. Go into a situation intentionally un-aligned, off-balance and find your balance as you play the game, that's where the honey-hole is, where you're most alive.

I still ain't forgave myself for not getting you that college application in time. I didn't think you were going to get shot so soon. I mean, we all got shot, it's like a black eye growing up on Rock Creek Church Road. It's the "Caveats of Hustling." If you can't take a bullet or two? I suggest you go do something else brudda'.

Furthermore, I didn't think you and Quack would succumb to your injuries. I promise with every cell in my body, I'm sorry bruh'. I wish I could've taken those shots for boff' of you. This is not a form of self-deprecation but as man. I'm not a third of what you guys were. The world will know your name.

Anthony Johnson, aka "Diesel, the self-proclaimed King of Washington D.C. You walked it like you talked it brudda'. Rain, hail, sleet, or snow. If you want smoke? It's gunna' be a barbeque (colloquialism) no surrender, no retreat. e fight "till the death. That's just how it waz'.

You know I wasn't going to forget about you. If I hadn't grown up with you, we wouldn't have been friends. I told you that and you got maaaaad. But I thank God every day for having met you while you resided on the corner of my street. You made me tougher. Even in adulthood, when I had a difficult day in the ER and I needed to fight, not a treadmill to relieve my stress.

I will come and find you. We would fight for hours and then shake hands and buy each other a shot. You always kept it real and never ran when it was time for combat. I'm sorry I wasn't there for you when you crashed out. I had to tell your provider to take you off the ventilator. You had a traumatic brain injury crisis. Your pupils were not equal, round, nor were they -reactive to light and accommodation. A sign of papilledema and brain edema.

You had no blood flow to your tibial or dorsalis pulse; I wasn't going to let you become a vegetable, with no brain-wave activity. How you die at thirty-something after banging all them years? I did what you would've wanted me to do. I let you be free and get your Angel wingz. You're a distinguished angel now. God did an amazing job on you. From a knuckle-headed kid to a king. You did your job here on earth. I'm proud of what you accomplished. You did the best that you could. Most importantly, you wanted to see everyone else around you win. Although the feelings were not mutual. ~GodSpeed

Aim High Push Hard

Acknowledgements

God and his disciples, the universe for?!? You know what? Screw it, let's set precedents, not follow tradition. It's a new day. I would like to acknowledge spending time alone and not enjoying the company of my friends or family. It was a healthy constructive practice for me because there is only one person we are stuck with in this life.

To my young readers, I would like for you to stick with it, don't pull the parachute in discomfort, it will work itself out. The monkeys on your back will finally start playing and swinging in the trees and it will get organized. Because if you pull out too early when you're not getting along with yourself, it's going to bubble up in awkward ways later on and you're going to be forced to deal with the pain in other ways.

Kids aren't afraid to fall out of a tree, until they actually fall. So how high on that limb do you let them go, until you say, "No, no, no, no, no, because if they fall, they may fracture a bone or scrape their arm and receive an abrasion or avulsion fracture.

However, falling builds character, or maybe they won't fall! Let them negotiate situations for themselves. Let them negotiate decisions on themselves. Where does the want meet the need and the need meets the want? We have to figure it out. I got so many more results, when I didn't give a damn about the results. ~*GodSpeed*

Aim High Push Hard

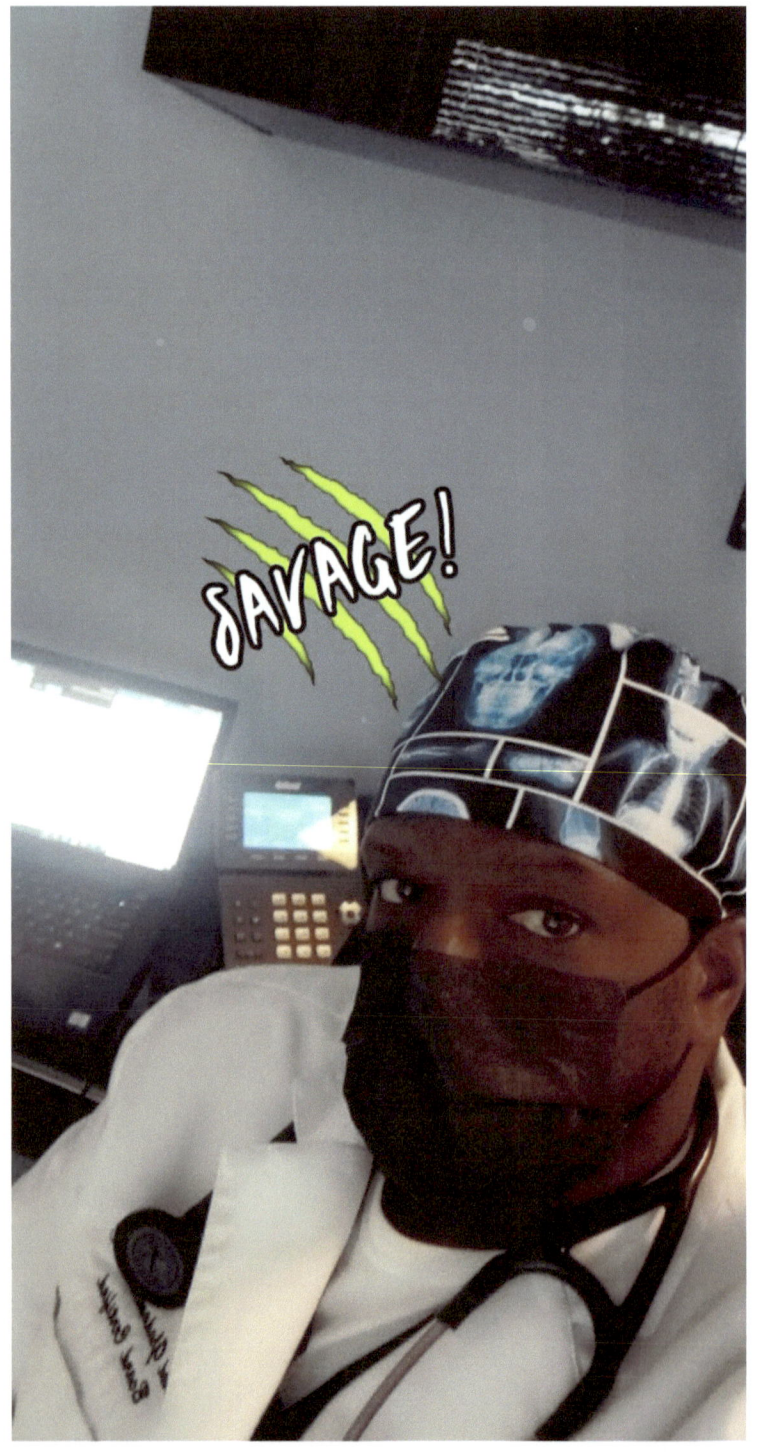

About the Author

I have no skeletons in my closet that can't be allowed out. Just because someone tells you that you can't do something, doesn't mean you have to listen. In Steve Jobs autobiography. His dad was a welder, who once told him, "Whether you're making a cupboard or a fence? You have to make the back of the cupboard or the fence, that no one can see, just as polished as you make the front. That way it will show your dedication and commitment to your work." This statement resonated profoundly with me. I approached this book in a similar fashion.

In this book, I let my brain get reconnected with my heart and soul. People need purpose, identity; People need something to cling on to. This book is what you will cling on to. I did not hold back on my trials or tribulations. This is a continuation of 17 CRIMES. Learn how a knuckle-head kid made it out of the ghetto to become one of the best Physician Associates in the United States of America, without a father figure, role model or guidance. I learned from my mistakes as I went along and didn't complain once. My mother is the truth, in physical and spiritual form. That lady tough as nails. However, a woman can't raise a boy to become a man. ~*GodSpeed*

Instagram: @aimhighpushhard

Twitter: @aimhighpushhard

YouTube: @aimhighpushhard

Preface

This is Book #2. A Continuation from Book #1, 17 Crimes. If you were remised in reading 17 Crimes? You won't understand this book. My aim is to write untraditional books. Different verbiage and a tad-bit different vernacular, because that's how I speak. My own books. My own life. We all have a ghetto-story. Well, here's mine! Enjoy it! A brother made it out of the trenches! Thanks to God. Lord knows I prayed a thousand nights. No embellishments and no fabrications. Now, how real is that? ~GodSpeed

Contents

Dedication……………………………………………………………………..i

Acknowledgements…………………………………………………………ii

About The Author……………………………………………………….…iii

Preface………………………………………………………………………..iv

Chapter 1- From Confinement to Commitment……………………..1

Chapter 2- Incarnation to Incarceration……………………………..14

Chapter 3- Adjusting to Change………………………………………29

Chapter 4- Finding My Way……………………………………………44

Chapter 5- No Matter Where You Go There You Are……………..59

Chapter 6- It's Always All Good Until It Isn't……………………….72

Chapter 7- High Speed Chase…………………………………………..89

Chapter 8- Central Booking Intake Center………………………..108

Chapter 9- Final Mulligan……………………………………………..115

Chapter 10- Metamorphosis…………………………………………..124

Chapter 11- Residency #1……………………………………………...134

Chapter 12- Residency #2……………………………………………..148

Chapter 13- Residency #3……………………………………………..167

Chapter 14- Graduation………………………………………………..177

Chapter 15- Board Exams……………………………………………..181

Chapter 16-Conclusion…………………………………………………186

Aim High Push Hard

Page Left Blank Intentionally

Chapter 1

From Confinement to Commitment

When I stepped out of those prison gates towards the end of August. I stretched my arms wide, looked up to the blue sky and let the sunshine percolate through my brown face. I yelled to the sky, at the top of my voice "Thank you God, I have been rehabilitated, reinvigorated, reassimilated and finally ready to be relocated; Virginia State University here I come. I was filled with excitement. I pictured the possibilities of making it big and all the fun that it was going to be.

"Ahmed, Ahmed." A loud voice shrieked as the voice broke me out of my ornament, as I was enraptured in deep thought. It was the last person I'd expect to see at this very moment. My mom! Mrs. Kilani and I sprinted towards each other and hugged as if we had never seen each other before. She said "boy, you shot up in there huh? You're taller than me now! You got strong too, what were you doing in there?" I simply replied, "Metamorphosis Mama." She said "Metamorphosis, what's that?" I replied, "It's a book I read in my cell by a man named Franz-Kafka. It was about a salesman, named Gregor Samsa who wakes up one morning to find himself inexplicably transformed into a huge insect; subsequently struggling to adjust to his new condition."

Mrs. Kilani replied, "So what are you trying to tell me Ahmed? That you're all of the sudden going to conform into a super-human creature to help eradicate your struggles?" I replied, "No, Ma, it's deeper than that, you just don't understand." She replied, "I'm your mother, the only thing you're going to conform into is a scholastic achieving college student and your most formidable struggle will be Advanced-Placement Calculus; You heard what the Judge said? This is it for you Ahmed! One more time and you're headed to the big house, where you have no choice but to rumble with the wolves, in order to survive." I replied, "Mama, I heard what she said, and trust me when I say, I have no intentions of ever going back to jail again. I wouldn't wish that place on my worst enemy." She replied, "That sounds like music to my ears."

Aim High Push Hard

As we entered the vehicle, I asked "Why didn't you bring Fela with you? Don't tell me that my little brother is too shy to see his big brother?" She replied in an ominous tone, "Ahmed, you broke your brother's heart on his birthday. He waited all day for that damn phone to ring and not once did your conceited ass call." I yelled aloud, "Conceited? You have some nerve; do you think I want my little brother to hear me talk about how I'm passing time in jail confined to my cell for 23 hours a day? huh? Caged in like some fucking animal?" "Ahmed, I'm still your mother, you watch your mouth when you're speaking to me young man." I continued "Sorry Ma, but another man telling you when you can shit, shower and shave? Heck no, I didn't want my little brother hearing jail stories. I did that time by my lonesome, like a man is supposed to do, and each day was like a living hell, taking steps to bring me closer to embrace a premature death. I went in there a boy Mama; I came out a man. Now, can you take me around the 'hood and let me say good-bye to the homies before I haul my tail off to college, please."

Aim High Push Hard

Mrs. Kilani said confidently, "Nah' ain't no more homies, I packed all your essential items, we are headed straight to Virginia State University and here is your first semester college schedule. 18 credits per/semester should be more than enough to keep you busy. Your first class begins promptly, at 8:15am, we better get a move on it." I sat back in the passenger seat and tried vehemently to conceal my displeasure. The exuberance of just being released from jail, coupled with the idea of going away to college was now fleeting. If I'd just had an opportunity to see Fela, give him a hug and let him know that I was sorry for letting him down, would have made a world of difference to me.

I now became ambivalent with the whole idea of this college thing. I didn't expect everything to happen so imminently after being released from jail. I had no time to process my emotions or to prepare for the formidable battles that lay ahead. I felt alone at a time when I should've felt solace, because I was finally going to be around the people that care about and love me. I felt as though I was just being cast-away to an isolated island like Tom Hanks, in the critically acclaimed movie *"Cast Away."* I couldn't gather myself to explain to Mrs. Kilani that I was having doubts about whether I was equipped with the mental fortitude to take on such a huge commitment. At the age of 17? I was still trying to figure things out about myself and wondering if I was as mentally prepared as I thought I was. "**Doubt**" began to creep in my mind.

The ambivalence became so prevalent in my mind that I began to reconsider the idea of this whole college journey. Self-sabotaging myself, cogitating things like, "I'm going to be a nobody in college. Everyone knew me in my hood, I considered myself somewhat of an authority figure, I had friends, family, I was comfortable in the hood. Outside of going to class, what would I do in order to keep myself occupied? What subject will I major in? Who will I befriend? Who will I study with? I should just go back to the hood, accumulate my money, buy a business in the neighborhood and integrate vertically. But a business like what? All I know is how to sell eight-balls, quarters, halves and kilos. What the hell am I going to do? Other than be a devil-filled dope peddler? I ruminated on the enumerate thoughts so much that it gave me a tension-type migraine headache.

As I reclined the front passenger seat and let my feeble body sink into the leather seats, I slowly drifted off to sleep. When I awoke, I couldn't believe my eyes. Mrs. Kilani said emphatically, "Wake up, we're here, wind your window down and look around you Ahmed, isn't this beautiful?" I replied *"Hellllllll Nooooooo,* what in the holy-grail heck is this." All I saw were trees, grass, and long dirt roads. I thought I was dreaming and landed back in Africa, so I pinched myself on my left forearm to ensure that I wasn't. And sure, as the skies are blue, I was living in reality.

I figured I would do my best to make the most out of a culture shocking situation. I felt like I was sinking in quicksand. I looked around and marveled at all the other college students of different ethnicities, who spoke different dialects, and wore different styles of clothing. It was all so confusing for me to wrap around my mind. I felt like a fish out of water on hostile territory. I only knew how to deal with things one way.

Suddenly, I made an outburst to no one in particular, stating, "If a dude plays with me out here like I'm a country-bumpkin, I'm taking his head smooth off of his shoulders like Jeffrey Dahmer."

Unbeknownst to me, the emotions that I was experiencing were an ***"adjustment disorder"*** to my new surroundings. Which is characterized by preoccupation with the stressor of culture shock and failure to adapt to a new situation. The predominant feature is a disturbance of conduct that leads to a feeling of inability to cope, plan, or continue in the present situation. I was also experiencing ***"generalized anxiety disorder"*** Which is characterized by preoccupied thoughts of worry, impending doom and despair.

What a 17 year/old young man hasn't realized is that these are all normal behavioral patterns of a mammalian human-being, hoist from a concrete jungle, where chaos is a normal way of life, into a controlled setting without being ***"deprogrammed."***

Aim High Push Hard

"Deprogramming" is a vital tool that all inner-city high schools need to incorporate in their course curriculum and assimilate in the students that are in the eleventh and twelfth grade year of high school. This is necessary in order to prepare students who endured hardships and have yet to develop the necessary coping mechanisms to function in a controlled learning environment.

He or she must learn how to detach themselves from the feelings of paranoia that comes along with having foreign people around them on campus, wanting to hug you because that is the primary form of greeting and displaying signs of affection in their culture. In Washington D.C. where I grew up, if you look at someone to long on subway, they will shoot you in your head. These are adolescents that we are speaking of. It isn't right. We have to create a viable solution.

Furthermore, I believe that teachers who choose to rule with an iron fist, that won't hesitate to lock the classroom door if you weren't punctual to class needs to be revised and repealed as well. I'm not saying that impunctuality should be tolerated but teachers should emphatic and bear in mind that these kids come from tumultuous households, where the hour between 1pm and 2pm is breakfast time for urban youth where you can usually find us at "waffle house" ordering a patty-melt with the hash browns, salt and pepper, ketchup. In all seriousness, teachers shouldn't lock the classroom door. The alarm clock that young boys have been conditioned to in the inner-city to wake up is when their cell phone rings for their first sale of the day.

Another method of ***"Deprogramming"*** is how teaching kids that utilizing the same conflict resolution tactics that helped you survive and maneuver your way through the neighborhood's concrete jungle to solve disputes with other students and professors could get you expelled from the university that could potentially be your gateway to a bright future of financial freedom. But who was I kidding? This was the Commonwealth of Virginia, where typical neighborhood words like ***"bitch", "muthafuckas" "fuck" and "shit"*** words that were a large part of my vocabulary during my childhood, were all met with a swift misdemeanor charge of: ***"Use of Vulgar Language,"*** which was punishable by up to six months in jail and a $5,000.00 fine. I can't blame my mom for that! She never utilized that type of language. She spoke with stellar vernacular and was always at work trying to provide and support to put a roof over our heads, whenever she came back from Nigeria. I take full accountability and blame myself for hanging out on the corner after school, where thugs, pushers, pimps, and prostitutes were my daily dose of social assimilation. I learned to ameliorate my social skills later on, but the damage was already done. The punishment received from my transgressions was severe.

I knew from my previous run-ins with law enforcement to stay on the right side of the tracks and all, but, how the holy heck did they expect me to just know some off the wall stuff like that, straight off the top of my dome? **Mental telepathy? Clairvoyance?** I mean, give me a break!

The **"Deprogramming Phase"** should last no more than a duration of three months, six hours a day; Five days a week, with a break in between each segment. I mean, we don't want to bog the kids down with modern day cliches. We just want to give them a *"real world"* etiquette view from an impoverished perspective. It all boils down to whether the kids want to work sedulously and study voraciously, ascertaining information to become perspicacious and give it a 110% in order to be capable of reaching their full potential. Thus, earning the dreams that seemed further and further from the clasp of their hands, with each drive-by murder of one of their childhood friends.

Similarly, the **"Deprogram Instructor"** must be exceptional at transcending the information they are trying to get the student to engage in. You can't just speak from experiences that are not your own. It doesn't come across as sincere and it damn sure isn't genuine, the kids and students will take notice of that façade and resent you for it.

Let's just stop kidding ourselves! We all know that having the opportunity to obtain a collegiate education is a privilege in this country. But if you have a certain demographic of colored children, whose parents and fore-fathers help architect and build this country through toiling soil, blood, sweat, whips, and tears. Still, they paid taxes to this country and they, themselves, were victims of circumstances that were out of their control because of the measures that they, themselves, had to take to escape the perils of poverty! Wouldn't you marvel at that child for overcoming formidable obstacles as you would marvel at a rose that grew from concrete with jagged edges, thorns and withered petals? This rose could have crumbled a long time ago, but it chose to flourish and live out its true faith, changing the world, one mist of aroma at a time.

That is the object of **"Deprogramming"** urban kids and students, from just one summer course. There is no college orientation that can match that level of maturity and precociousness, In that short of a time span. That is how you level the playing field for disadvantaged urban youth and enact change in the process for a bright future. We must give these kids a chance, otherwise we risk losing them to the streets for good. Unfortunately, once the streets have an alluring vice grip on your kids, they never come back the same. They are forever tormented and irretrievably broken. Spiritually? They are gone asunder, and there isn't any coming back from that. Not without cognitive behavioral therapy. And even with that the chances are slim to none. Slim just walked out the door. Electroconvulsive therapy may be the only reasonable solution but then you risk acquiring retrograde amnesia.

Chapter 2

Incarnation to Incarceration

I was walking to the Virgina State University Cafeteria one day and spotted Big-Ant, a 7th-N-Taylor crew member. I chased him down like a red nose Pitbull chase down the mailman delivering mail at high noon. Big-Ant, who was over 6ft' 3" and weighed over 300 pounds. We both played on the same football team, in Washington, D.C. in 9th grade when I attended Roosevelt Highschool before being expelled. He played offensive tackle. I played running back and when we locked eyes, he took off running, like he played running back. The entire school was out there chattering to one another, "Who is that guy chasing Big-Ant across the school cafeteria?

Big-Ant eventually stopped running in the middle of the cafeteria, after he saw security guards who became alert to the situation and said "Man, we're in college; we're supposed to leave all that beefing stuff in the hood." I said "Whaaaaat, nigga, you got it aaaaaallll wrong, your homiez shot my brother and that means that we're beefing in the past, the now, and for the rest of our lives." Big-Ant's face turned to a flush bright red color as if he saw a ghost. Security quickly took note of the malicious encountering that was about to transpire before their eyes in a college cafeteria and deescalated the situation. I roared "You must be about to go from offensive tackle to playing full-back the way that I'm gon' have your scary ass runnin' all 'round this campus, this isn't over!" I went back to my dorm-room and laid down for a second to gather my thoughts. Saying to myself, "Maaan, I need to go back to the crib and get my bread just in case some stuff goes left out here." Unbeknownst to me, my visceral intuition was speaking to me.

    I waited until Friday night, that way I would have completed all my classes and have most of my homework done. The rest of my unfinished homework, I planned to work on while I was on the greyhound bus. I had to take the greyhound for the first time in my life. It was a full bus-ride, set to depart promptly at 9:00pm. Crammed with people of all ages, genders and ethnicities. The ride was from Petersburg, Virginia to Union Station, in Wahington, D.C. It was going to be a long, arduous, trip, but I wasn't willing to allow myself to lament over it. I fell asleep as soon as I got on the bus. The greyhound bus ride was rather peculiar to me. It kept making multiple stops, taking repletes during the trip to disembark and then embark riders along the journey; Making stops in places such as Raleigh, Charlotte, Durham, and Fayetteville, North Carolina. I suddenly realized that I was on the wrong bus because I was supposed to be headed back towards D.C. and not North Carolina. Talk about being a bone head!

    I jumped off the greyhound bus in Fayetteville, North Carolina and then hopped on the correct bus to Washington D. C's Union Station. When I arrived in D.C. I went straight to Mrs. Kilani's house and grabbed the stash of cash and immediately went back to Union Station to get on a greyhound bus back to school. I didn't want to risk making any false moves that would lead to me going back to the slammer. When I arrived at the house, I searched every room for Fela before I left for Union

Station, but low and behold, Fela and Mrs. Kilani were nowhere to be found, so I left without seeing them and having the opportunity to say goodbye, which was disappointing and unnerving for me. During one of the stops on the way back to Petersburg, Virginia, I went exploring through a used car dealership and purchased a '96 Nissan Maxima. Now, at least I had some wheels to go to the grocery store and stock up my fridge in my door-room because I was sure enough tired of eating at the school cafeteria.

On September 12, 2001, I went to algebra class. I happened to have a professor, who was of Pakistani descent. I didn't mind the cultural differences; I was there to learn but I couldn't have chosen a worse day. On the infamous day that planes, hi-jacked by terrorist crashed into the Pentagon in Arlington, Virginia and the World Trade Center in New York City, simultaneously. In a lighthearted manner, the algebra professor segued from the course curriculum and began asking the class questions about how they felt about the tragic incidents that transpired a day prior to class.

Aim High Push Hard

One of the questions he asked the class was, "What would you all do if you saw Osama Bin Laden?" I quickly raised my hand and answered in a jokingly manner "I would prob'ly try to kidnap him until I received ransom money from his folks to release him. I would also try to kidnap you while I'm at it; Call it a 2 for 1 special. if it guaranteed that we wouldn't have to take the mid-term exams!" The classroom burst into a heaping laughter. Everyone, including me, thought the joke was right on the eye and funny, none of the students took offense to it. Unfortunately, the algebra professor did not share the same sentiment. Being as though, news channels were broadcasting planes with passengers on board were hi-jacked by Afghanistan's and Pakistani's. The professor didn't think the joke was too funny. I extrapolated this from the contemptuous look on the teachers face. His fiery eyes piercing back at me was enough for me to realize that this was far from over, and the Pakistani algebra professor would seek retribution against me.

Nonetheless, the bell rang, and class was dismissed. I breathed a huge sigh of relief just to be able to get out of there, the tension was thick. I decided I had enough for one day and would head on back to my dorm-room, grab a quick bite to eat and do some studying before heading off to bed early that night. But I couldn't sleep that evening, I tossed and turned all night. Something about that professor and the way he kept scathing at me during class didn't sit right with me. I began to question in my mind, what did the tattoo that the professor had on his hand symbolize? Was it some homeland cult? Or maybe a representation of honor? Did he think that I was trying to make a fool out of him in front of everyone because that was not my intention, I was simply being facetious, but you know what they say? ***"The road to hell is paved with intentions."***

      The next morning two law enforcement officers from Petersburg County, Virgina knocked on my dorm-room. **Booom Booom Booom!** I awakened in a stupor, stumbling to the door, I hesitantly opened it and there were two scrawny 6ft '3, 250Lb white men in police uniform at my door. One of the officers stated, "You mind putting some clothes on?" I replied, "For what?" The officer stated, "We need you to come down to the station with us." "What am I going down to the station with you guys for?" The Officer stated, "Your algebra professor elected to press charges on you for making a terroristic threat." I said "That's bull crap. I was only joking with him, and he knows that." The officer said "Well, young man, you can tell it to the judge." I quickly began considering all possible outcomes and how I may not be released on my personal recognizance, due to my lengthy criminal history. I said to the officer, "give me a minute to put on my clothes. I need to grab sone money just in case things go left and I need to bail myself out of jail."

    I gathered myself and proceeded to exit the room as I asked, "By the way, is the Petersburg, Courthouse handling this case? It occurred on university property; shouldn't this be handled by the school's security department? The officer said, "Well, if the teacher filed a complaint to school security, then maybe. But he didn't! He pressed charges against you down at the Petersburg, County Courthouse. Come on, let's go, we're taking a ride to the police station, don't worry, you'll be back shortly." As we drove to the jail processing center. I had an eerie visceral feeling that things were not going to turn out in my favor, but I remained optimistic. I was glad I grabbed a roll of money from my dresser drawer, which was just under $6,500.00.

I arrived at Petersburg, County Jail and it was certainly unlike any place I've been incarcerated in. For starters it was in the middle of nowhere and it took us an hour to drive there. It was off a beaten, dirt path road, tucked in a cul-de-sac, between two wide cornfields. This entire experience was rapidly becoming a disaster, but I would have to lace up my boots and face this head on.

When I walked into the jail's processing center, I noticed the hallways were much longer and narrower than the previous jail I was in, and the inmates were segregated by race. Thus, congregating only in their section and with their ethnicity. You had your *"Aryan Skinheads,"* your *"Muslims"*, your *"Black Guerilla Family,"* and the *"Vatos,"* whom all, made up much of the prison gang population. Oddly enough, I noticed through sheer observation that the Mexicans seemed to have the most structure amongst them. They only answered one individual who was known as the **"Head Honcho."** I figured if things were to go left and I had no choice but to stay and do time, I would have to get close to the *"Head Honcho"* but that certainly wasn't the outcome I hoped for. I was simply preparing myself for the worst.

After going through the intake process. I couldn't understand why I was placed in the general population with other inmates who were doing football numbers. It wasn't like I killed anyone, but I was in a unit with violent offenders. Some had 7 years, others had 14, 21, 28, and 36 years to life. I asked the correctional officer, "When do I see the commissioner so I can have my bail hearing and get the heck up out of here?" The correctional officer replied, "They'll call you when they get ready for you so grab yourself a snicker candy bar because it's going to be a while." I then replied, "The officers told me that I was just coming in to get booked and I'll be out shortly." The correctional officer said, "Look, all that is between you and the judge, keep it moving."

At this point, I was incensed beyond measure, but I remained calm because I knew my bail wouldn't be more than $60,000 for a misdemeanor. I understood the law enough to know that it wasn't uncommon for a bail to be set that high for a misdemeanor charge. Especially when dealing with the Commonwealth, of Virginia. I quickly did the math in my head and figured at 10% that would be $6,000 and I can get myself back to school and back to class. I thought they would confiscate my money when I was booked in, but they let me keep it on my person. I transformed back into survival mode once I entered the jail dormitory-hall. Of course, all eyes were staring at me as if I was fresh tuna and the jail inmates were sharks waiting to attack. But I wasn't tripping off them and figured I'd break the tension by *ripping a major fart* right in front of everyone, **Brrrrrrump...**

    One of the *Aryan-Skinheads* said, "Damn, man, what you got a trumpet back there?" I replied sarcastically, "Nah, it's a saxophone, you want to see if you can play a note?" The *Aryan-Skinhead* didn't know how to take that response, so he just said "Whatever." I gave him a menacing look up and down before going to lay down on my bunk. I made that joke to provoke him into a confrontation, so I could get the fear of thinking what if someone tries me in here out of my head. " If other inmates smell fear, they prey on that weakness, and you become a victim. They take your money, bed mattress, commissary and even your soul if they think it's vulnerable enough. Some inmates even go as far as making you pay taxes for the cell that you sleep in as part of the cost for coming into their prison, as if they own it, it's incredulous."

I don't care what anyone tells you. Prison, jail and detainment centers, are all *"**Wack as hell.**"* You never get reformed from being institutionalized. Instead, you become coarse and develop a vehement, vindictive vendetta against society and everyone in it. I understood that I had to be punished for my transgressions in society to maintain law and order. I just didn't agree with having to be locked behind bars in a cage like an animal to drive that point home. Being incarcerated is dehumanizing in every aspect. After twelve hours of impatient waiting, my name was called to go see the commissioner for a bail review hearing. Before leaving my cell, I was shackled; wrist to feet like a slave by the guards, only able to shuffle my feet a few inches at a time. I said,

"Damn C.O. all this for a joke I made in class, this is a tad bit excessive don't you think?" The correctional officer replied, "Welcome to the Commonwealth of Virginia."

At the bail hearing, I sat in front of the commissioner and was made aware of my charges, which were, ***"Threating to Do Bodily Harm."*** A class 1 misdemeanor, punishable by up to 12 months confinement in jail and a fine of not more than $2,500. The commissioner then imposed a $60,000.00 bond. That was surprising to hear but I understood that in this country, African Americans pay two to three times as much in penalties and monetary fees, i.e., attorney cost, fines, court fees, and probation cost than our Caucasian counterparts. Apparently, the cops turn a blind eye because the Caucasian kids are viewed as innocuous and non-mischievous. The cops also reside in the suburbs and not in the inner-city where they target colored people more frequently because that's where the government chooses to allocate most of their funds to add additional officers who are not from the same ethnicity, thus not being able to resonate with the young black male's plight. These officers sometimes live three to four hours away. How can they be in tune with the pulse of what is going on in the trenches? *"The System Is Rigged"*. I'll let you use your judgement and ponder on who it's rigged against? And who's doing the rigging!

Furthermore, bearing I could post a bail of 10%, or use my home as collateral, which I didn't have because I resided in a freshman dormitory. I asked the commissioner, "Do I have any other options?" The commissioner replied, "Yes, you can remain incarcerated until your arraignment hearing in 30 days. I shook my head left and right, before mumbling, "I just got out of jail, I can't stay here for thirty days and risk flunking my first semester of college, not to mention the Judge in Washington, D.C. theoretically dug me out of a hole when she furloughed me from jail early to pursue my academics, and here I was again about to throw it all away. When will I learn that if I keep learning the wrong lessons, I'll continue making the same mistakes. I have no one to blame, other than myself.

The commissioner snapped me out of my trance when she retorted "Young man, what was that? I can't hear you when you're mumbling." I said, look, "I have $6,000 in my pockets right now, can I give it to you and get back to campus, I really need to pass this semester. People like me don't get second, third, fourth and fifth chances in life; can you grant me some leniency?" The commissioner, flabbergasted, replied, "You have $6,000 cash in your pockets, right now?" I replied, "Did I stutter You George Washington looking muthafuckah? and went into my right jeans pocket to pull out the money. But the sudden jerk of me reaching into my pockets to pull the bail money out caused the links in the handcuffs to squeeze even tighter into my skin, causing paresthesia in my hands as a result of my bilateral radial and ulnar artery being compressed. I was finally able to pull out a wad of money rolled in a rubber band of 6- $1,000 stacks. I said "Okay, here it is, "One, Two, Three, Four, Five, Six, now take these bracelets off of me and let me free!"

I was visibly upset at myself. I hated the act that I couldn't seem to stay out of trouble. It was as if no matter where I went, trouble would always be there to rear its ugly head. But again, I wasn't **"Deprogrammed."**

Chapter 3

Adjusting To Change

When I was released from Chesterfield County Jail in Petersburg, Virginia. I called a cab. When the taxicab driver arrived, I hopped in the backseat and said, "get me the heck away from here as fast as you can, I never want to see this racist place again."

The taxicab driver was a big-burly man in his late fifties.

The cab driver replied, "I reckon by your accent that you're not from this neck of the woods?"

I said, "That's because I'm not, I'm from the city. If we're speaking veraciously, other than enduring jail, adapting to this place is one of the hardest things I've had to do in my life."

Aim High Push Hard

The taxicab driver replied, "Life is hard, it's mean, it's unfair and treats you worse than a cantankerous mistress." He then continued speaking, "Son, the world can be so cold that it chews you up, swallows you whole and spits you out. One must have the ability of an amphibian to withstand the fire that life throws your way. The people who withstood the flames, come out the other side rising from the ashes, like a phoenix. Unaffected and stronger than before, after all, what doesn't kill you makes you stronger." Old man was spitting game, so I sucked it up.

It dawned on me that he was speaking about my existential experience. How could he have possibly known what I was experiencing? Or what I was yet to experience?

The cab driver dropped me off in front of my dorm at Virginia State University. As I exited the vehicle he said, "Young man, before you get out, I will leave you with this, you are of age now, at a collegiate institution where they do not give a damn about how difficult your life was. They are only concerned with your academics, so you need to develop a set of different values and choose a metric barometer of success with how you measure it by."

I replied, "elaborate sir."

The cab driver proceeded, "Ask yourself, what is really important to you in life, your answer will be your set of values. Then ask yourself "why are these values important to me?" That is your metric barometer, that will be used to measure how much you believe in each value."

I replied, "So if I change my values will my problems go away?"

The cab driver chuckled before responding, "Life is all about problems son. With different values, come a different set of problems, but you will rather have good problems than have to endure the daunting pain from dealing with all the bad problems that life will throw your way." I understood every word he said and took it all into consideration. His words resonated with me profoundly. There are some conversations that people will have with you throughout your life's journey and God is using them as a vessel to speak through vicariously.

The next day as I walked into biology class, my cellphone rang and I answered it, "*Hello*" while lecture was occurring (I knew this was a huge no-no,) But again, my **"oppositional defiance"** began to fizzle its way to the surface. The professor said, "You better hang that phone up and sit your ass down." Everyone in the class burst out laughing hysterically. The **"oppositional-defiant disorder"** kicked in and I felt humiliated, so I squirted water into the professor's face and walked out the class.

The culture shock combined with dealing with **"adjustment disorder"** of having to be in a foreign place. Not to mention being quickly submerged into foreign waters; with crickets, birds chirping, roosters crowing! No streets, no corner stores, no blocks and the closest store was a Walmart that was twenty miles away. I wasn't sure if I had the willpower to do it anymore.

As I entered my dorm building headed for my room, I got a glimpse of my next-door neighbor's wall and noticed he had a "*RIP Lil Larry*" shirt hung up on his wall. I knocked on his door and walked right in and asked him, "How do you know Lil Larry?"

He replied, "That's my man, Pistol P, from the 1-4 zone."

I replied, "*Oh yeah*! He used to knock dudes down on 5th and Kennedy Street. They would run and hide under the car whenever he pulled up and he would get out of his car and leisurely walk to the car they were hiding under and shoot underneath the car. Until they scattered like roaches or bled out like a stuck hog. Then he would come up to our hood and show love to all the homies. Lil Larry was a real good brother man, it hurt me to my soul when he was murdered." And just like that we bonded. He said, "My friends call me Mally."

The next day I had my case hearing, I went to court, and I was astonished to see all thirty of my classmates and Algebra professor in the court room. One after the other, they took the witness stand to attest to the fact that I indeed said those words to the professor. The judge passed a guilty verdict without giving me a chance to speak on my behalf. I was asked to pay a fine of *$2,500.00* and sentenced to twelve months in jail with all suspended but one day. The whole class started clapping their hands and cheering. Being experienced with the law due to my recent unfortunate run-ins with authorities, I knew there would be no jail time because twelve months was suspended and the one day, I did at Chesterfield County jail ,, in Petersburg, Virginia would suffice as time served.

After the court case, I met up with some of my classmates. Just out of curiosity, I asked, "What's up with that? Why did you guys testify against me?"

One of my classmates retorted, "The teacher promised to give us all an **"A"** in the class, if we testified against you in court, but we have nothing against you. What you said was funny. I didn't think you meant any harm by it, but this is a commonwealth state, and any small infraction can be considered as grounds for expulsion.

I was so confused because I could not fathom a life where people do things to demoralize someone else for beneficial gains.

Although I had good grades in all my classes, I could not help but get into mischief on campus, like the time when I began sipping soda from the soda-machine fountain in the school cafeteria and spitting it out because it tasted flat. Subsequently, I was charged with "*grand-larceny, theft under a $1,000.00.*" Or when the midget looking school security officer kept giving me this ominous look as I was chopping it up with Mally on campus one day, while we waited for class to begin. I stared back at him with my right fist balled up in my left palm. I was charged with **"threatening to do bodily harm,"** taken to the campus security office and was given a citation to return to a college disciplinary hearing before I was released. I had a litany of allegations against me, stemming from gambling for money, rolling dice with classmates during class, after completing my assignments and being overcome with boredom. The professor said to me, "You will never make it anywhere in life, shooting dice during class, you're going to end up on the street corner, lying in front of the liquor store begging random strangers for change."

Towards the end of the semester, in December 2001, I had a 3.8 GPA. I was elated because it was a stressful semester, but I did not have time to relish the moment because I was called to the Dean's office. He asked me to take a seat, I knew I wasn't about to hear any good news by his callus demeanor.

He began to speak, "Due to all the incidents that has occurred during this semester, we will have come to the conclusion to expel you from our program."

I replied, *"Wait A Minute!* I have a 3.8 GPA, what do you mean "expelled?" That's quite excessive, don't you think?"

The Dean replied, "Yes, you are one of the brightest students at this program but there are just some behavioral issues you have going on in your life that need to be addressed."

I replied, "Look you are not my dad so spare me with all of that fatherly advice. If I must leave school, that's one thing, but an expulsion on my academic record means that I will be precluded from applying to any other colleges, because collegiate institutions do not accept expelled students. Is there any way that you can keep the expulsion off my college record?"

The dean acquiescently obliged before replying, "Yes, but only on one condition.

I replied, "What's the condition? I'm all ears."

He retorted, "you have to be banned from entering the state of Virginia for a year as well."

I replied, "One year? Why do I have to be banned for a year? It isn't like I assaulted, sold drugs, tortured, or killed anyone."

The Dean replied, "I know it's a bad rap, I'm not trying to be your father. But from a black man to another black man, those red-neck white boys up in Chesterfield County. In Way over yonder in Petersburg, Virginia do not want you terrorizing their state."

I replied harshly, "Terrorizing? Who are you calling a terrorizer? What do I look like a member of the Klu Klux Klan? Because they are the ones who galivant around the United States dressed in patrol uniform after they leave their rally for the *"Let's go Nigger hunting campaign."* annually. It gets swept under the rug as a *"good 'ol boy convention"* I further exclaimed, "I'm a black college student struggling and striving, doing my very best to keep my head above water in Amerikkka, playing the cards I was dealt, and I was dealt a shitty hand from jump street. Let's be clear, I'm not looking for pity, but I would like for you to empathize with my situation and life stressors." I felt dehumanized, and the dean was beginning to display a lack of empathy, while going on a tirade defaming my character, which really got under my skin and began to unnerve me in all veracity.

I walked to my dorm room, packed up all my belongings and caught the next available greyhound bus back to Mrs. Kilani's house.

Mrs. Kilani was furious when I told her about the school's decision, which I expected. She's a fiery Nigerian woman, one who does not mince her words. She yelled, "You are not going to stay in this house; not for six months. So, you had better start applying to other colleges." I recalled the conversation I had with the taxi-driver about developing a set of different values for myself. I began to think, "I value education because I want to be knowledgeable, and my academic performance will be my metric barometer used to measure my success." I had an important decision to make, I did not want to go too far from home, and I also wanted to be in the city. However, I knew I couldn't let cognitive dissonance settle into my mind, thus causing me to become conflicted by being faced with opposing arduous choices and choosing neither of the two, thus being rendered helpless and opting to do nothing at all. It can be viewed as a form of self-sabotage and that is not beneficial for anyone. With that in mind, I was able to nail it down to two options: Howard University or Morgan State University. I chose Morgan State University because Howard University was too close to home and being too close to home is a recipe for disaster. I projected enough self-awareness to realize that I'd be up to mischief in no time. Subsequently, I applied to Morgan State University and was accepted with alacrity.

One night, Fela, G-Y, Bullet, Moose and I, along with a few other friends were all chilling at Unc's house on Manor Street in Washington D.C. playing John Madden football on a PlayStation gaming console for $400 a game, when the *"ATF"* suddenly knocked the door down with a battering ram, which startled me. Fela began crawling across the floor trying to get to the bathroom in a hurry to flush his stash down the toilet, he stuck his hand down the commode, and I was right behind him, simultaneously pressing the handle to flush the toilet and it all went down the drain in the nick of time. Sweat began to trickle down my brow as we scurried back into the living room where Moose had just thrown his stash underneath the sofa and Fela sat right on top of the stash. As The *"ATF"* came into Unc's house in full riot gear one of the officers said, "So, this is where you guys have been hibernating during the winter huh? No wonder we haven't been seeing you guys posted up on the corner of *Rock Creek Church Road.* What? Is the weather a tad-bit too nippy outside for you hustlers to work your corners suddenly? I know you dudes aren't going soft because of the cold weather and minor wind chill, is that why you dudes are hiding in this house?" All the *"ATF"* members burst into synchronized, sarcastic laughter. It was low down, shameful and pathetic, if you ask me. *"ATF"* officers, making light out of a terrible situation. The only way to describe it in layman terms is a nostalgia of going back to when we were kids playing cops and robbers; well, I pretty much felt like the robber that got caught. I snapped out of my ornamental deep thought and composed myself.

G-Y replied, "Hiding? We don't do any hiding."

One of the *"ATF"* officers replied, "I'll tell y'all what, since y'all like playing John Madden football video games so much, I'll play one of you in a football game and if I win, I haul y'all to jail."

Moose replied, "What happens if we win?"

The officer said, "Then you all get to go home, unless something illegal turns up inside here while we're searching, then everyone goes to jail."

Moose replied, "Fuck it then! Let's get on with it, there's no need to talk about it, take us to jail, it's not as if it's my first time going to the slammer."

Aim High Push Hard

I replied, "*SheeedN'me*, I'm on a respite from school, I'm not trying to go to a white man's private prison, doing manual labor for 0.25 cents per/hour. I just dug myself out the grave by re-enrolling in college, it's a miracle I was accepted, because most people aren't granted a second opportunity at academic achievement. I don't want to ruin my opportunity of becoming someone in life, again." They continued searching everyone meticulously, until they serendipitously stumbled across car keys in each one of our pockets and pressed the car alarm to each car and searched the corresponding vehicle. Talk about bad luck combined with bad timing. They didn't find anything but fingerprints. After searching for another hour and a half, not finding anything, they grew weary and left. That was when it hit me, I said to myself, "This is not the move, I'm not giving up school and potentially what can be a great future to come back to this. It was as if the signs were all there, I just couldn't read them, but God was speaking to me loud and clear. I couldn't decipher what he was trying to say to me, but I did feel this supernatural clairvoyance coming from him. As if God was using him to speak to me and tell me everything that I needed to hear. The way that God speaks to you sometimes is bewildering. God uses people, places, things, emotions and punishment (although God is merciful) to speak to me. However, I felt confusion, perplexity and cognitive dissonance. I didn't know which way to go but I knew I had to move, staying still would've killed me in more ways than one way."

Chapter 4

Finding My Way

When I arrived at Morgan State University I felt at home. East Baltimore, it was like a rundown version of Washington, D.C., forty-five minutes to an hour drive away from the nation's capital. That meant it was far enough so I would have to think long and hard before making a two-hour round-trip drive back and forth to D.C. Although I wasn't used to all the "yo-yo-yo" slang of the Baltimoreans, I conceded in the fact that I felt liberated and was able to do what was needed in order to succeed and graduate on time. The only dilemma was that I didn't know what degree I wanted to major in. Medicine was on top of my list but due to all the injustices I witnessed people of color go through combined with the plight and the social ills of the ghettoes in America I felt compelled to choose social work as my primary major.

My first class of the semester was Introduction to social work, the lesson of the day was on **"Why social workers are overworked and underpaid?"** The professor explained, "Not only do social workers have to make house calls, link citizens with 28-day drug rehab programs, initiate their insurance coverages and get them housing. On top of all of that, they are also responsible for being a liaison or a conduit for people from disadvantaged backgrounds to obtain decent employment." I thought to myself, "*woo,* that sounds like a huge commitment"! Doubt began to rear its ugly head into my world. You know what they say about doubt? You must annihilate it or else it consumes you and erodes your core from within indolently, until the habits that doubt creates, i.e., distraction, video games, watching television, random lascivious sex-capades with multiple partners, gambling, scrolling for hours on social media, looking at the same negative images, and procrastinating on achieving your goals, becomes too big of a chain to break away from. Now let's break it down deeper into a scientific compound. These things further create a physiological response. i.e., high blood pressure, fast heart-rate, muscle tension, sweaty palms, dilated pupils, increased heightened immune response system alert, which makes you susceptible to opportunistic infection." All these things are a culmination of a recipe for disaster and sudden cardiac death from the sheer stress alone.

The professor proceeded, "After a year of working grueling hours, providing altruistic services to America's low socio-economic class citizens, do you all know how much we take home?" Before the class could make a guess, he said, *"$29,300.00 per year."*

I raised my hand and asked, "How much does a social worker make with a Ph.D.?"

He replied, *$39,500.00 per year.*

I said to myself, "I don't think this is the major for me". I want to dedicate my life to public health services, but not at the sacrifice of what I deemed as a weak financial ceiling, after all, this is America, where the cost of living is high, and inflation increases at 3% annually. I have to be able to sustain the cost-of-living expenditures. Subsequently, I changed my major to Psychology. I've always been fascinated by the intrinsic human mind and how it works, and I figured I could draw from my troubled past to help me relate to patients with mental illness, thus promoting a better mental space for the patients that I treat. In Psychology 101, again, the topics discussed were salaries. I began to realize that college was a business due to all the monetary lessons that I was initially being taught.

    The professor stated, "Choosing a career as a psychologist is not an easy task. The emotional strain we endure from being a mental sponge, absorbing patients' pessimistic views, the patient on physician violence, working days, evenings and weekends. Most psychologists spend many years in isolation, combined with the expensive education and training required. Do you know how much we take home annually? $44,000.00, if you get a Ph.D., you can make anywhere from $50,000.00 to $70,000.00." I said to myself, "I could manage that, but the question still remains, will I be fulfilled with my career choice?" I decided to go back to my dorm room and mull it over a bit.

Aim High Push Hard

As I entered the building, I got off the elevator and began walking to my dorm room. I noticed two boys shooting dice in front of my dorm room. The sheer gull, and audacity of them to *"shoot craps"* at a collegiate institution and in front of my room was flabbergasting. One of the boy's names was Beazy, a real down to earth, introspective type of guy. I thought it was disrespectful to shoot dice in front of my room and I wasn't going to ask them to move. Instead, I walked right through their crap game, stomping the sole of my dirty shoes all over the dice money, with no contrition. The same way that "Rick James" the singer stepped his muddy boots all over "Eddie Murphy's" couch back in the 80's. Beazy said, "Damn 'cuz, you can't say excuse me? I looked at him eye to eye and said, scathingly, you excused." Beazy shook his head in disbelief before saying, "This dude is wild, he must be from D.C.?"

I heard that and replied, "Uptowns finest, don't get it tangle and twisted". For some reason, I just could not let that hood mentality go. Even when I did my best to suppress it. It would always rise to the surface like grits, boiling in a creamy, hot crock pot. As I laid down on my bed, my stomach began rumbling so I went to the bathroom to take a boo-boo. When I got in the stall, I noticed a fresh can of lemon Lysol spray sitting on top of the commode. I said to myself, '*Oh yeah*' the angels are all around me today wanting to make sure I don't pick up any crabs or some other transmittable disease that could jump from this toilet seat on to my black behind. It was four dorm rooms on each floor and two students in each room sharing one bathroom. I finished my bowel movement and took the can of lemon Lysol back inside my room.

Two minutes later, there was a knock on my door. *Knock, knock, knock...* "Who is it?" I shouted.

"It's Beazy, your next-door neighbor," he replied.

As I opened the door, I sarcastically said, "Look, I don't have a microwave that you can borrow so don't come over here begging, cause I ain't lending you none of my stuff, black people always needing something."

Beazy retorted, "Microwave? Nigga, you tripping. I have my own microwave."

I incessantly replied, "So, what can I help you with?"

Beazy asked, "Did you see my can of lemon Lysol in the bathroom just now?"

I said, "Lysol?" I then walked to my computer table and picked the can of Lysol up to hold it up in the air so he could see it and stated, "Are you referring to this can of Lysol, which is complimentary for the freshman dorm bathroom, yeah I seent' it. I thought I'd hold on to it in my room for safe keeping. I don't want people using it up all *Willy-Nillie*."

Beazy retorted, how are you going to ration out my can of Lysol? Man, if you don't give me back my Lysol." I respected him from thereafter because he stood up for himself and didn't just let me bully him and take his Lysol. So, I gave the little nigga back his can of Lysol disinfectant spray. We chalked it up to a misunderstanding and Beazy stated "I'm from Suitland, Maryland. It borders the south-eastern part of

Washington D.C. I wasn't too familiar with Maryland, but I heard about Suitland, Maryland a time or two. Majorly, because NBA Basketball player *"Kevin Durant"* went to Suitland, Highschool in the 9th grade. I heard through the grapevine that Suitland, Maryland was one of those places in Prince George's County, Maryland that can instinctively give someone a sense of false security because they think it's one of the richest counties in America until someone walks up on you and tells you to alleviate your pockets, robbing you of all your belongings. Things can turn from sugar to manure just that quick in Suitland, Maryland.

    Beazy and I subsequently developed a stalwart friendship. Through Beazy, I met some more dudes from Maryland like Corey aka *C-Moe*. A real basketball talent in Highschool. He played point-guard for Charles H. Flowers and planned on walking on the Morgan State Men's Basketball team. He had a sweet jumper with a soft touch, ~ala~ *"Isiah Thomas"*. But, when you hoop and smoke weed, it diminishes your respiratory drive, causing you to fatigue quicker than the guys on your team, as well as the guys on your opponent's team who don't smoke cannabis. Some people can smoke weed and hoop, without any negative effect on their game whatsoever. *"Kevin Durant"* is one of them, *"James Harden"* is another, but most people can't.

He also introduced me to Perry aka *P-Stat*. He coined himself P-Stat because he "stayed on his own status." Perry was a highly ambitious journalist, with a passionate opinion on everything. He had an uncanny knack for instruments and sports reporting. He played keyboard for a prominent go-go band in Washington D.C. called (T.C.B) Total Control Band. They were decent at getting the go-go parties "turnt-up" in the area, but I wasn't into go-go parties, it wasn't my thing, so I stayed clear of it.

Then, there was Marcus. His demeanor reminded me of myself, the previous year, when I matriculated at Virginia State University. Marcus was "**Deprogrammed,**" rambunctious, and ready for whatever. He was a year younger than me so I figured this would be a great opportunity to redeem myself in the eyes of the most high, for my past transgressions. Thus, taking Marcus under my wing and making him my protege. I began schooling him on the college *do's and don'ts.* Albeit I wasn't acclimated to all the college *do's and don'ts* myself as I was just beginning to plant my feet in fresh cement. But I sure was up for the challenge.

Our mundane activities consisted of going to class, consuming cannabis together during the interim and playing video games. Lots and lots of video games. Ironically, I played more video games in college than I did when I was hustling (Go Figure!). You spend a lot of time by yourself in college and more time in your dormitory room when you're living on campus, so you have more people to play video games with. The only contrast was that we weren't waging any monetary odds on the video games, to me? that was futile, but when in Rome, you do as the romans, so I played the video games during my down time and focused on my studies for the majority of the time. I figured I was now doing things the right way. Since I was in college, why not partake in toking a little gunja? Unlike, former president *"Bill Clinton"* who admitted to smoking cannabis but fibbed about inhaling it. I, on the other hand, happened to take a toke of it, *inhaled it, and liked it, yes, I did*, it helped me to relax and prioritize objectives that I needed to complete in an organized and timely manner. I made a mental note to cultivate cannabis in the future for the medical benefits.

I began to take a more meticulous approach to course curriculums and the classes that I was taking in order to ascertain exactly what I was committing myself to. I was able to deduce that most of the courses I was taking for a psychology major would be deemed transferable to another university, with the addition of a few core classes. I would be able to apply to Pharmacy school in two years, without having to wait patiently for a 4-year degree. I discerned that college was a stepping-stone to finding a suitable career. A career that was brimming with lucrative qualities.

Studies have shown that an inordinate amount of college graduates are displaced into job sectors that they dislike. Largely in part to them being unable to apply the knowledge they acquired from their tedious college education. Furthermore, they are underpaid to the point where they have no other alternative but to move back into the ghetto that they came from because of the cost of living is affordable there, however, the constant violence is free, which is why you hear about college graduates being murdered in the neighborhood that they grew up in. That defeats the purpose of working sedulously to receive a college education. I refused to spend every dollar I had on my college tuition only to graduate and work at *"Women's Footlocker"* selling the patrons who patronized the store, sneakers and pumps for the rest of my life. Henceforth, I also was not there for the college fraternity experience, it didn't appeal to me at the time. It still does not appeal to me now. It's a distraction, especially in your first 2 to 3 years of college, it's a major distraction that derails you and sidetracks you from what you went to college for. It's great if you want to get into the alumni fraternity or sorority chapter after you graduate school but if you're serious about your academics. In my experience, I would hold off on the pledging situation.

Aim High Push Hard

Precociousness and Impetuousness are two of my most formidable weaknesses. I equate it to being too smart and too fast for your own britches. You end up making an enumerate quantity of mistakes that way, thus ending up paying hefty fines for it, which all aren't monetary. Some fines cost you to lose sleep and others cause unyielding stress levels.

Albeit I was blessed with the ability to be a philomath and capable of grasping concepts quickly when I was exposed to subjects and foreign topics. My drive to climb the ladder of success and not follow the traditional four-to-five-year graduation plan was something that unnerved me a great deal. The self-doubt that consumed me of whether I could really pull this off began to creep into the **pre-frontal cortex of my frontal lobe.** Nevertheless, I **annihilated doubt with alacrity** and **persevered**, full steam ahead. I decided to load up my courses to 21 credits per/semester, which was unheard of at the time. I believed that it would allow me to **complete the prerequisite courses for Pharmacy school, while simultaneously pursuing my Psychology degree.** I coined it a "two for one special." College wasn't going to use me for my school tuition, leaving me in debt for the rest of my life and dumping me into a nursing home or on the side of the road at a homeless shelter after it was finished with me. It has happened to many Americans, and I wouldn't allow it to ail me. I planned on being perspicacious, as an astute student and utilize college to my personal advantage.

One day on my way *to Cell and Molecular Biology Class.* I stopped dead in the middle of my tracks and asked myself, "Why do I really want to be a pharmacist in the first place?" I then ruminated upon the thought "Is it because I have a strong proclivity to sell drugs?" The answer to the question was a conundrum in my mental that left me feeling vexed.

When you can, always ask yourself, ***"If you want to do it, before you do it?" Because, if you don't want to, you're going to do a half-ass job, which is equivalent to doing nothing at all. The result is time wasted, which is not an asset.*** *Wasted time* is merely a liability and life's too short to be a jack of all trades and a master of none. You just don't have the luxury to be proficient at multiple things in life.

Aim High Push Hard

Yes, I knew my way around manufacturing, marketing and distributing various drugs. But I loved learning the pharmacological mechanisms by which opioids relieve pain and induce euphoria when crossing the blood-brain barrier and accessing the central nervous system where its effects begin to manifest. I also had a yearning to learn about antibiotics, HIV and Cancer medications so that I could help eradicate diseases in the minority communities across the United States of America.

Chapter 5

No Matter Where You Go There You Are

While I passed all my exams with flying colors. I couldn't help but notice, Beazy getting major paper. I mean **Majorly, and I wanted a piece of the action**. I wasn't pocket watching or anything. No, I was merely taking reconnaissance of my surroundings and I saw an opportunity present itself.

During one of my mundane-mindful walks from my dorm room to my classroom, students would always stop me to inquire on whether I knew "Who had the weed for sale?" For the sake of my life, I couldn't conjure up why it appeared as though students and just people in general would always make a beeline towards me in droves to ask for cannabis? It wasn't like I walked around reeking of marijuana or advertised anything of the sort. Maybe it was the dreadlocks hairstyle I monikered that gave me away. Or maybe it was my apathetic demeanor? At any rate, they knew, that I knew, who had the *"za's"*, that's what we called exotic marijuana in my hood.

    I saw Beazy walking to class one day, and I calmly asked him, "Hey man, do you think you can bring me back an extra pound of cannabis when you go back home to Suitland, Maryland this weekend?" Now, I don't get me wrong. I could've gone right back around Rock Creek Church Road and got a Pound of cannabis to distribute for a cheaper number than what Beazy was getting his for. But my pride wouldn't allow me to go back to the hood and hear people say, "Man, you in college and still selling drugs? I thought you were walking a straight and narrow line?" Naw, Naw, I didn't want to hear that narrative. Or even be enticed to come back around the hood and hang out with the homie because it would have made me comfortable and jubilant. Again, I came too far but the devil was always lurking on my back, just waiting for me to slip so he could take over my soul, and I wasn't allowing it. It was hard ya'll.

Beazy being a *quid pro quo type* of individual replied, "SheeedN'Me, what's in it for me?"

I said, "In it for you? You're already grabbing two pounds every weekend for yourself, just bring your boy an extra pound back."

Beazy retorted with alacrity, *"Exactly! I'm bringing two pounds back to sell for myself.* If I add a pound, then I'm incurring extra risk, if I get pulled over and arrested by the cops will you come and bail me out?"

I gave him an ominous gaze before replying, "You're being dramatic and paranoid for no reason man, stop what you're doing. *Aaaaain't* nobody getting pulled over and *Aaaaain't* nobody going to jail, don't manifest those thoughts or they may come into fruition… But I'll tell you what I will do! I'll buy you a full tank of super unleaded gas, premium octane '93 gasoline. You're going to be driving until next year with that super-unleaded, premium gas. It doesn't burn like regular unleaded gas. It's like the *energizer bunny,* it just keeps going and going and going."

He said, "Cut the jokes, you must plan on riding with me too then, huh?"

I replied, "If I could, you know I would with the quickness. Unfortunately, I have books on top of books that won't read themselves. Don't fret though; I won't forget the favor." Beazy acquiescently complied and drove down to Washington D.C. on a Friday night. He returned to Morgan State University two days later, on Sunday night, with three pounds of the *"za's."* I threw him *$1,150.00* for the pound and broke it down into ounces *(28 grams a piece)*. I sold each ounce for *$200.00*. They were all gone before my first class on Friday morning. I grossed *$2,050.00* profit. A total of *$3,200.00* in revenue. I added *$250.00* to the *$3,200.00* and threw Beazy *$3,450.00*. I told him $to bring me back three pounds this time and I was off to the races from there. The business scaled vertically and the *"za's"* practically sold itself on campus and in the dormitories, without me advertising it. What marketing? That would've proved futile. If you find a product that sells itself? You ain't gotta' market a damn thing. Does Bentley market their vehicles on Super Bowl commercials? I think not!

I always wondered why all those New York and New Jersey dudes, like Zig who never graduated college were still galivanting around campus on a routine basis as if they were lions waiting on a gazelle to pass by them so they could jump on them. I thought Zig and his cronies just like the freshman girls and couldn't get enough sex. They were all well over 30 years old. But as fate would have it, the boy was wrong. They were there selling *"za's."* That was their career choice, Zig and his cronies were indifferent about attending a *Historical Black College University, aka (HBCU). The sweat, tears, bloodshed, death and sacrifices that our ancestors had to make for us to be blessed with an opportunity to receive an education in this country. There was once a time when African-Americans were castrated if we were caught trying to learn how to read.* However, they were determined to sell dime bags until the apocalypse came or the school shut-down, whichever came first. People are going to live their lives however they choose to, and that's their prerogative, it's just the way they go about doing it that is inexplicably abhorrent to me. But hey, who am I to judge? I have a cup full of sins and I live in a glass house so it would be unfair to throw stones.

The following day I was in chemistry class when engineering students walked from their building to buy cannabis from me, which was quite a distance across campus to the pre-medical students building. They would wave at me to come into the hallway. I wasn't taking any chances and motioned for them to meet me in the bathroom. I waited until my chemistry professor offered us class intermission to meet them in the bathroom, sold a couple of ounces and went back to class to finish up the day's lab experiment. I was no longer defiant, nor did I disrespect the professors. Not even a joke was made in class. You didn't hear a peep out of me, unless it was to answer a question that the professor asked me. That jail stent I did at Chesterfield County in Petersburg, Virginia **Got my mind right.**

When class ended Beazy, and I would meet up and go to lunch. We stopped to pick up Corey after his class ended and headed straight to

Red-Lobster in Towson, Maryland. Beazy and I ordered the *ultimate feast platter*. Which came with Maine, steamed-lobster tail, crab legs, shrimp linguini, loaded baked potato and all you can eat cheddar bay biscuits. These were not your ordinary cheddar bay biscuits. These were the cheddar bay biscuits that taste so **darn-goooooood,** they make you want to slap your *Mama*. We then washed it down with Red-Lobster's, strawberry-lemonade that tasted as if Aunt Shirley was in the kitchen churning strawberries and lemons with her feet and hands to make it. I could taste the sweetness of the strawberry cut perfectly with the bitterness of the lemonade in each sip. *Talk about a five-star meal in a two-star restaurant*! I wasn't complaining, that's for sure. Compared to the microwave food that we had to take from our dorm rooms to reheat in the cafeteria to eat? **The ultimate seafood platter from Red-Lobster back in the day? Laaaawd have mercy! It was an umami, delightful, savory-dish. As I'm writing this book now, my mouth is watering for them cheddar bay-biscuits.**

Now, Corey on the other hand; He ordered water with lemon. When the water came out this *foolio* had the nerve to say some ol' cliche stuff like, "when life gives you lemons, make lemonade." I snarky stated, *"SheeedN'Me,* you might want to add in a few packets of *Sweet'N Low* to make it taste a little sweet, otherwise, *that's a bitter life."* As Corey added the *Sweet'N Low* to his water and squeezed the lemon slices over top, he began to stir the water around in the glass. Beazy and I vehemently tried to keep from laughing but we just couldn't help it and burst out into synchronized laughter.

Corey's feelings were visibly hurt by us poking fun at him. I could tell by the disgruntled look on his face.

I said, "Stop laughing Beazy. C-Moe, what do you want to order? I'll pay for it; the waiter is coming." He stated, "I'll have the chicken fingers and french fries, with salt, pepper, and a side of ketchup."

Again, I tried to hold in my laughter, but I couldn't resist. I blurted, "Man, where do you think we are? McDonald's? You're ordering a kid's meal? Would like a toy with that meal too? With a large McFlurry?" I teased him further, "Beazy where did you find this dude?"

Beazy said, "Chill Ahmed, Corey is cool, he just has to learn the ropes." I replied, "he needs to learn how to keep shooting that basketball to improve his jump shot. "*Slanging*" packs is not the ropes he needs to ascertain."

Corey said, "True, but I don't want to keep ordering chicken nuggets and fries while ya'll feast on crab legs and lobster tails."

I replied, "Well Corey, you can always eat in the school cafeteria, it is covered under your room and board expenses, you know?"

Corey countered, "nah, I'm good. That food tastes horrible." We all finished our food before heading back to Morgan State University to attend the remainder of our classes for the day.

After class, I walked to my dorm room to get some rest. When I got to my building and pressed the elevator button to go upstairs, I heard some nice sounding instrumental beats at the perfect octave level coming from one of the dorm rooms on the first floor, so I followed my ear to the sound and knocked on the door. A 6'0 feet, light-skinned guy with cornrows opened the door and said, "What's up?"

I replied, "What's good foolio, are those your beats in there bumping like that?"

The guy responded, "Yeah, I do a little something from time to time."

I retorted. "You make beats? That's Cool, do you mind if I come in there and lay down a verse to that dope ass beat that you just cooked up? I can feel the flames coming off the cords. I'm gon' murk that beat, one take, stop playing."

He said, "You rap?"

I replied, no, but I have a lot of pain I need to get off my chest. This might just be the cathartic release that I need."

He stated, "Bet, my name is Ricardo. I'm from the city!"

I replied, "Oh yeah, me too, what part of the city are you from?"

He said, "Southside, come on in my studio, I'll play a few tracks for you, and you can jump on whichever one you like."

I jumped on the first track I heard and laced all three verses with precision. One take and I was done. Ricardo said, "Damn, you rode straight through that beat, didn't you? Did you already have the verses written down or something?"

I hesitated and thought about my answer long and hard, before responding, and thought back on my life before exclaiming, "Yeah man, it was written. God wrote my life a long time ago. I just drew from the experiences that I've encountered throughout my life's journey. I feel relieved. Thank you for letting me get that out of my system."

Before I left, I said, "What type of name is Ricardo for a musician as talented as yourself?" We should shorten it to "Doe boy." Yea, that's a fly name right there. You digging that my guy?"

He retorted, "Yeah, that's cool."

I asked, "Do you have a band or is this just a hobby?"

He said, "I just started a small group called Blood-Brothers Entertainment, you're more than welcome to join us if you want to?"

I was flattered, but I did not want to take it seriously, pursuing it full-time because I knew too many stories of starving-artists. In my mind I extrapolated that I'd wind up another aspiring famous rapper **"*frustrated, famous, and penniless*"**. I just needed to release the pain that I repressed since childhood, however ambivalently, I didn't want to decline Doe boy's offer, so I said, "Let me ruminate on it and I'll get back with you after class tomorrow with an answer." Doe boy replied, "bet that up my guy."

The next day I attended class, then went right back to Doe boy's dorm room to record in his studio. I finally felt a feeling of belonging because I found an extra-curricular activity that I enjoyed doing in between classes and people who I enjoyed doing them with. Walking to class and back to your dormitory room everyday can quickly become monotonous and cause depression to settle in. College no longer seemed like something I had to force. Every existential experience felt natural, like I was living a normal life. The more I rapped, the more pain I released. There were a lot of emotions to unpack, which caused me to yell ferociously on the microphone while recording most tracks. When I finally recorded a record about where my future was taking me. I became more optimistic, and my world began to open wider; I no longer felt myopic-minded, it was sort of like I was manifesting my own destiny and shaping my life. Unbeknownst to me, words have power, and I was beginning to project the words I spoke into reality. Every rhyme I wrote began to come into fruition. I'd be remiss if I failed to mention that it was one of the best times of my life. I said to myself, "Man, I could really get used to this college life, with a big ol' Kool-Aid smile on my face, from ear to ear. Everything was working. I felt better than I ever felt before. I just had to let go and let God deal with it. You'd be surprised how God laughs at our plans, while we are busy planning them. That's usually when life happens to us!

Chapter 6

It's Always All Good, Until It Isn't

I left Microbiology class after a sixty-minute lecture on antimicrobial agents, Methicillin-resistant staphylococcus Aureus. As I walked back to my dorm room to study for my next exam. I entered my dormitory; I noticed some people shooting craps on the back stairwell behind doe-boy's room. Prince George's County boys versus Baltimore City boys. I figured, what the hell? Let me jump in and win some money quickly. **A funny thing about gambling is, you always think that you're going to win but never stop to consider the factor of losing everything you own. Everyone likes to be in the know. Even when we lose two and win one, we believe in the one more than the two. We believe the number we roll that hits big was a product of our truer selves, was when we met our potential and read the future, was when we were gods. The two losses, however, were aberrations, misfits, glitches in our** *masterminds, even though the math clearly makes them the majority. Nobody kn-owwws who is going to win, there is no sure thing, that's why it's called gambling. There is a reason Vegas and Reno continues to grow. They kn-owww we bettors love to believe we do. That is a lock.*

The minute I jumped in the game, I began to lose two and win one. Marcus was gambling, winning, throwing numbers, left and right he couldn't miss. Derrick was side betting. I figured it wasn't my night, so I decided to side bet with Marcus, betting on all the numbers that he rolled out. I began winning all my money back, so I took another shot at the dice and started throwing passes. Number after number. Seven and eleven was all a brother was throwing. Then I rolled the dice again and went smack out. Craps, shoot, I lost!

One of the Baltimore dudes said, "Yo, these D.C. niggas sweet yo." I replied, Adamantly, "If you're not gambling, please do me a favor and shut the fuck up." I knew he wasn't gambling because he had no money in his hands. He subsequently ignored my stern, vehement warnings and kept on running his mouth, further antagonizing me.

Aim High Push Hard

I did the dumbest thing that I could think of. Which was, letting my emotions overshadow my intellect. I got up and said to everyone, "I'll be right back." Marcus picked up the dice and started gambling. They didn't have any suspicion as to the anger I foolishly allowed to slither so clandestinely inside my young mind as they proceeded to gamble. I went to Doe boy's room, which was just a few feet from the crap game and knocked on the door. Doe boy opened the door and was ecstatic to see me as he cheered. "Man, I was just about to call your ass. I just made this fire ass beat that I want you to flow on.

I said, "later for that music shit Doe. Where your banger at?"

He replied, "In the glove compartment of my car, outside in the parking lot. Why, what's up?"

I anxiously replied, "Give me the keys!"

Doe said, "Ahmed, man, holla at me, tell me what's going on?"

I felt like Doe wouldn't understand my emotions and what compelled my anger to surface but that was my ego and pride, which wouldn't allow me to explain it to him. I already made my mind up about the events that would soon transpire. I felt violated by the Baltimore dude calling me "sweet" albeit, he wasn't directly calling me sweet per se, because he was generalizing about the entire urban population of Washington D.C. and just teasing me to get underneath my skin. Looking back on it, it worked. I let my ego get the best of me. As I write this book at this big age. I'm aware that there may have been some miscommunication, misinterpretation and emotional immaturity occurring. Doe said, "here you go, take the keys."

    I snatched the keys from his hands and walked out of his dorm room. As I walked down the long hallway. Frank, from Prince George's County, walked past me. We were always cordial with one another at school and would greet each other when walking on Morgan State's Campus bridge. We both had a visceral feeling that one another was from the city when we met. But we never spoke past saying "wassup and goodbye." It was a "real recognize real type of vibe that we had for one another." A mutual understanding of respect between two black men without having a friendship. When someone is really from the trenches, you just know. They don't have to walk around broadcasting it to everyone like a newscaster. You just know, that's all.

Frank said, "Ahmed what's up man, why do you look so upset? I shook my head, ignoring his question and kept walking. Again, the male ego compounded with pride exuded its ugly head, permeating my humiliated soul.

Frank said, "Ahmed, whatever you are about to do, just know that it isn't worth it bro." I slowly shook my head from side to side.

I clenched my teeth and put my grey hoody over my head before slowly turning my head in an ominous manner, back over my shoulder, looking Frank sincerely in his eyes. There was no conceding on the inappropriate decision my mind conjured. Once I make up my mind to do something, I'm fully committed and dedicated until I see it through completely. There is no contrition, only retribution.

Aim High Push Hard

The sincerity in Frank's tone of voice resonated with me vehemently. I thought for a split second whether it was actually worth it or not to kill these Baltimore city boys? My plan was to shoot boffum' in the head one after the other and watch the blood ooze from their skull and be filled with jubilation. In that instant I reverted to my old ways. On the verge of losing everything I worked sedulously for, to rob some dudes with low wages that made me feel played. I couldn't let them get away with disrespecting me in that appalling manner.

I felt like *"my name was my name,"* and if I allowed my dignity to become compromised, I felt as though my honor and manhood would also become compromised and the comparable feeling to describe it to is similar to growing up in an impoverished community already plagued with danger and having a Caucasian police officer who isn't from the community dehumanize you by calling you abhorrent words like ***"boy"*** and ***"nigger"*** *then beat yo' ass in front of everybody. They're aware* that you can't do a damn thing about it because they have pepper spray, rubber bullets, real bullets and batons, so you grin and bear and accept it. But this time I was the *"rabbit with the gun"* and an ineffable power came over me that I cannot put into words. But if you've experienced it before, you're familiar with the surge of adrenaline combined with rage that will make the most gregarious black man catch a murder charge on the humble all because he feels the need to demonstrate properly on another person. All the while I was acting off emotion. Not being cerebral. Allowing someone else (no matter the color of their skin) to have power and control over my emotions, to make me do something so heinous that it could land me in prison for the rest of my life! Just thinking about the buffoonery, I allowed myself to go through makes me unnerved.

Could you possibly imagine that I never once stopped to think to myself and say, *"Hey Ahmed, what if they have weapons on them and shoot you in the head?"* or *"What if one of them wrestles the gun away from you and kills you with it?"* I never pondered any of those options as possibilities. That shows you how irresponsible, careless and juvenile I was still behaving in college, still living life without guidance making mistakes as I went along. You don't know how many times I prayed for a father to speak to. A man who's been through what I went through and could help relieve the mental torment and pressure that I felt. It was a travesty but with every test there is a testimony. I wasn't going to sit there and lament over it.

I got to Doe boy's car and looked inside the glove compartment. In there was a 38cal. handgun with only one bullet inside the chamber. I had a decision to make. **A) Put one bullet inside the circular six round chamber and pray that it squeezes off and I hit my mark (Headshot!) Or B) Just run inside there, bare face and pistol whip the fuck out of all of them? I chose the ladder because it would be more efficient and drive my point home. They needed to feel my pain repressed from all these years of trepidation. Trepidation from my peers and the police, I finally boiled over and reached my tipping point. That was the final straw.** I hopped out of Doe boy's car and gangsta walked my ass all the way back to the dormitory hallway. I reached the end of the hall, at the back stairwell and kicked in the door where we were all previously gambling with my left foot, and said, "Lay all of that shit down, my trigger finger has a proclivity to twitch when I'm vitriolic. Matter of fact cuz' lay it down slow and don't make any sudden movements, get on the ground you all know what time it is, *Jackpot*." I said it, with a smirk on my face. Although I was upset, it was comical, you had to be there to understand it.

The irony is, I didn't even want their money, I wanted to humiliate them. The same way they humiliated me. I was immature, lacking emotional intelligence, and I had some serious self-insecurities that I needed to deal with, but I was unaware of what I was experiencing at the time. No one taught it to me, and I hadn't read the unresolved, repressed, childhood-trauma and behavioral health issues books yet. I couldn't control whatever anger that I was experiencing. I didn't expect Marcus and Derrick to hit the deck and spread their arms out wide like an eagle that had soared through the sky the way that they both did.

I walked up to the B-more dude that was talking all that smack and banged him in the head with the pistol. A huge dehiscence opened on his forehead, causing blood to splatter all over the adjacent wall in the stairwell. I turned and hit the other Baltimore dude with the pistol. He began leaking blood from his face, I needed to drill the nail home some more, be more sinister, be more malevolent, be more malice so the B-more dudes could adamantly understand the intensity of the violation that they committed against me. As I said earlier. I grew up in an environment where I watched people get shot for less on a mundane, routine basis, they had to feel my pain. So, I said, "Both of ya'll, empty your pockets, take off your shoes and clothes, strip-down butt-naked, ya'll gon' run home naked today, ya'll both gon' remember this day. I'm going to make sure it leaves an indelible memory on both your brains."

As they rummaged through their pockets emptying all the contents on the floor. Marcus and Derrick glanced at each other through their peripheral vision, and both got up and hauled ass in unison out of the stairwell, for some strange reason I was surprised by that, I assumed they were tough because they boasted and bragged about what they did in the streets as children **(Which I later learned were whole lies, they were good kids, who grew up in functional households, with mommy,**

daddy, grandl) unlike me. I now looked at them as wimps. I had the gun still pointed at both Baltimore dudes. After they took their shirt and jeans off, they ran as fast as they could out of the stairwell. I started laughing, little did I know that this was the beginning of a disconcerting night. I gathered all their belongings and went up to Beazy's room upstairs to tally everything up.

    I knocked on Beazy's door, he opened it and said, "What's up with you Ahmed?"

    I replied, nonchalantly, *sheeed,* just cooling, what you got going on?"

    Beazy replied, "Just up here playing NBA 2k, nothing much."

    I began emptying the B-more dudes belongings from my pockets to count the score. Beazy looked down at the pile of money, before hesitantly saying, "Damn, Ahmed, you been cleaning up, haven't you?" He was under the impression that the money came from the pounds of cannabis I purchased from him.

I snarky replied, "A little something, something. I just had to alleviate two Baltimore dudes of their paper and clothing for perpetrating like they were gangster's."

Beazy quickly flashed back, "Ahmed, you think that shit funny dawg? I got 2 pillows (pounds of cannabis) in here. Then you come back to my room with that shit possibly implicating me for something I had nothing to do with. What if they decide to retaliate? Did you consider that?"

I said, retaliate? Those college prep boy dudes ain't going to do nothing. I underestimated my opponent, 'cause it be the most scariest dude that'll pop your top out of sheer fear, without any contrition whatsoever. Beazy paused the video game and looked at me intently, before asking, "How do you know that them dudes you were gambling against go to this school?"

I replied, "Because their student I.D.'s are right here, duh!"

Aim High Push Hard

When I looked down on the bed, I realized there was only one Morgan State University school I.D. The other guy didn't attend the school. I slapped my hand down on the mattress, before exclaiming, "Sheeed, I thought they both went here?"

It's ironic, the broke Kermit the frog face looking one was the dude who had the most mouth, and he doesn't even go to this school. I figured he'd have some money on him. A food stamp card, Medicaid card, a red-cross card, just in case he had to donate his blood for money, anything. His wallet was hollow as an empty bottle of whiskey. Broke motor-mouth talking muthafuckah; he deserved everything he had coming to him. It's always the loudest ones in the room with the mute pockets. Another lesson learned!

We were both suddenly startled by the knock at the door. I clutched the 38cal. and whispered to Beazy, "make sure you look through that peep hole first, don't just swing the door open, you don't who's on the other side of that door?"

Beazy, "Sarcastically, replied, "Maybe you should've thought about that, before you decided to come up to my room after pulling a move."

I said, "man, whatever, niggas get braced everyday in my hood, open the door slowly, if it's them B-more dudes, I got one in the chamber of this .38 caliber revolver, Imma' just keep squeezing until it bust off, if he dies? Well, he just dies."

Beazy looked horrified after hearing my remarks. He opened the door, and to his surprise, it was Marcus and Derrick." I said, "Man where the fuck did you niggas run to?"

Derrick replied, "Sheeed, we got ghost man, I didn't think you were going to lay them bustas' down! I thought you were going up to your dorm room to get more money wo we could continue gambling."

I said, "Nah, sorry to inform you but, you got it wrong, 'cuz was talking too much smack and I figured I'd shut his broke ass up, that simple." But it wasn't truly that simple. My ego and pride were still in the tough guy, you have something to prove mode.

Marcus said, "Damn, I was just starting to clean them up too!"

I said, "Look, fuck all that sentimental shit, what's done is done. The Baltimore dude that I was gambling against had 4 grand on him, I'm about to go and invest that, buy some more *za's* that buy some more cannabis and sell it, at wholesale value to get rid of it quicker. I ain't holding on to no evidence stemming from an on-campus robbery. By the way, I found credit cards here too. The other dude ain't have nothing though. I'm about to go to the gas station and swipe these cards to the limit, fill my tank up before they call their bank and deactivate these cards." Looking back on it, I was so casual about it as if there would be no consequences to my actions. I wasn't thinking things all the way through, acting off pure emotion, not being cerebral. Challenges I faced all my life. The smartest people make the dumbest decisions.

Beazy said, "Nah, I'm good I'd rather stay in here and finish playing this video game. I'm not about to jump on that crash mission with ya'll. You niggas going to jail!" He screamed in a sarcastic tone.

I replied, "okay, suit yourself." As I walked out of his room, Derrick and Marcus followed behind me. When we got downstairs and exited the dormitory, I saw 20 niggas in all black walking through the parking lot. I said, "Do ya'll recognize them?"

Marcus said, "Yeah, I think that's them bustas' you just laid down for they paper."

I lifted the 38caliber. out of my right jean pocket and squeezed twice. Click, click, but no boom. The gun did not fire. The B-more dude I robbed earlier came back with a gun, I stared at him as he pointed the gun into the air, closed his eyes and let off one round. Then, they all dispersed. I squeezed the gun again and another click, with no boom.

"What type of old rusty .38 caliber handgun is this?" I yelled. The gun wouldn't bust off. I didn't care if I had one bullet or twenty *bullets*!

My life was in imminent danger. Whether I caused the Baltimore dudes to retaliate or not was inconsequential at this point. The war was on. It's so ironic how quickly sugar can turn into shit. One minute life is all jovial. The next it's filled with trepidation, and you were the primary cause of it. They say our lives are already written before we are conceived. I'm a bit ambivalent about that statement because I believe how we respond to certain stressors in life can alter the course of our direction in life.

Chapter 7

High Speed Chase

The twenty Baltimore dudes ran like they were at a track meet, although only one of them attended the university. I still pursued and chased them down, Marcus said, "Look up, the security camera is recording you, foolio'." I realized, if I kept squeezing the trigger and shot one of them on campus, the incident would be caught on camera, and I would be justly charged with an attempted murder charge. SheeedN'me, I wasn't that stupid to kill someone on camera, but in life, things don't always go the way you planned it. When you get jammed-up you really find out who your man's is.

I looked at Marcus, who was by my side and said, "Where the hell is Derrick?"

Marcus said, "Derrick got scared and hopped in a cab, and went home to Goodnow apartments. It's ten minutes from Hillen road." Without thinking, I said, "Okay, let's hop in my whip and meet Derrick at his crib."

Mrs. Kilani loaned me her 1995 Nissan Pathfinder, with the 5th wheel on the back and 4-Hi and 4-low-wheel drive, for increased traction when you're driving through the snow. I never drove it because I walked around campus and didn't need to drive to class. I let it sit in the parking lot and only used it for emergency situations. For some peculiar reason unbeknownst to me, I was dubious that this was the emergent situation Mrs. Kilani thought I'd be utilizing her truck in. A terrible snow blizzard made it almost impossible to get to class because of the icy roads and poor visibility. Maybe, but this diabolical gangsta shit here? Hell Nah! Ma dukes ain't going for that. She would've gone into a full syncopal episode and right into asystole if she heard anything about this. Good lord, I caused my mama so much pain, without her even knowing it. I'm sure that I caused her just as much pain with her knowing it. I'm sorry Mama!

To be honest, it was a tough road that I only made tougher for myself. I take full accountability for all my past transgressions. I was wildin' illegitimately.

When I got inside the car, I noticed the gas tank was on "E", I said, "Shoot, there isn't any gas in here, let's stop across the street at the Exxon and get some gas before we drive to Derrick's house." I took a pause to think to myself "Why would Derrick hop into a cab and go home without me?" It perplexed me. But hey, I learned through experience that it's always the so called gangster's that scurry off when they feel the pressure rise. Just a painful lesson we all must learn to live on earth with. People are not who they say they are and most times not who they appear to be. Everyone's walking around pretending, living in some **hyperbolic fallacy** that they conjured in their minds. It's confounding to say the least.

Marcus said, in a trembling voice, "But, but, what about them B-more dudes?"

"What about 'em?" I said casually.

Marcus replied, "What if they're riding around looking for us as we speak?"

I turned my head to the right, where Marcus sat in the passenger seat and said, "Man, you sound like a whole bitch right now, if anyone comes back looking for us? They're going to come back looking for me, not your stop-drop and roll ass, if I didn't know any better, I would have thought you were on fire the way you were rolling around on the ground." As I teased and laughed at him

Marcus sensed I was referring to him, taking money out of his pocket and hitting the deck. He was correct, I wasn't throwing any subliminals, I was speaking directly to him, and I would deal with Derrick later. However, I was disappointed at them both, because if the shoe was on the other foot, I would have had their back right or wrong. Later, when we get back to a safe location. I'm going to pull you to the side and say, "hey don't do that again, that's not cool, you could've set off a melee, we can get killed that way, that's not how I get down." But I'm not going to abandon you in the middle of a melee. He replied, "Nigga, I wasn't scared, I didn't want the Baltimore dudes to think I had anything to do with that shit, so I ran." This taught me a valuable lesson about dudes who scream out *"Gang-Gang," "Ride or Die," "Snitches get Stitches," or "That's my brother from another mother who I'd die for." No, the heck they won't ~~* **stop lying.** You must test dudes with pressure situations before you can define someone as a loyal person. In all veracity, loyalty is fleeting anyway. Respect lasts longer.

    I thought it was a bullshit response. Especially after he pretended to be the hardest gangsta in school. However, I let it go and proceeded to get us to safety. As I pulled into the Exxon gas station, I noticed a silver Ford Taurus with tinted windows driving towards us, in a slow fashion. Marcus screamed in a shriek voice, "That's them bustas' dawg, we gon' die, I can feel it in my guts."

    I responded, brashly, "Man, shut your bitch ass up you ain't got no guts and you damn sure ain't got no nuts. Better stop talking and recline your seat, in case they get to shooting at this car, the bullets can penetrate the window and not hit you in your big ass head, I've seent' it happen to dudes in my hood when I was little." Although I was incensed with Marcus and his frightening ways. I didn't want to see his head get hit with a bullet and the boy die in my car.

Oddly enough, the silver Ford Taurus drove past us, as we both reclined our seats. I said, "There is no way, that's them! you mean to tell me they had another chance to take a clean shot at us and didn't shoot?" I asked. Because if it were me and I had not one, but two opportunities to murder my opposition? The entire car would be Swiss cheese. Then I would jump out of my vehicle, walk-over and open the car door of the enemy's vehicle and shoot them again at close range so they wouldn't be able to testify against me in court, closed case.

If indeed it were those B-more dudes in that vehicle, then they were rooks and not cut from my cloth. *The pedigree that I'm cut from was taught to annihilate any and all opposition in broad day light or nighttime. We were taught by the Original Gangsters who we admired and looked up to as kids to always double-back at the funeral of the opposition that we killed and shoot up everyone that's outside. I don't care who's out there, the pastor and the person reciting the eulogy could get shot too. They shouldn't have been at the funeral of an active member, during gang conflict was the justification. No rules in war! It's always kill or be killed when growing up in a war-torn community.*

I still could not get over the fact that the little pee-shooter gun Doe boy gave me was a piece of shit, because I was still pulling the trigger towards the Ford Taurus, but the one bullet would not blast out the chamber. Abruptly, the Ford Taurus stopped at the intersection of Argyle Street and Hillen road, in Baltimore, Maryland. They proceeded to park on the corner but kept their headlights on.

I said to Marcus, "I have a visceral feeling that's the *"ATF"* foolio!

Marcus replied, "What makes you believe that?"

I said brashly, "Because dummy, they would've lit our stool pigeon asses up by now, and look how they are just sitting at the edge of the corner with their lights on as if they're waiting for us to pull out and pull off? My intuition keeps telling me that something doesn't seem right."

However, I persisted, stating, "If they're trying to be discreet, they sure are doing a lousy job." I listened to my intuition and jumped out of the vehicle and hid the .38 caliber revolver between the fender and back tire of the car that was parked directly behind us. I was 95% sure the car parked on the opposite end of the corner was the "*ATF*". My existential experiences learned from lessons that I was exposed to as a child taught me this. No soon as I wiped the gun clean, ensuring that my fingerprints would not appear on the gun in case things took a toll for the worse and the guys in the Ford Taurus were actually "*ATF*" agents as my intuition had insisted. Believe me, the last thing that you want is to be in court, going through an arduous trial and the prosecutor discovers the ballistic test came back with your fingerprints all over a weapon. That's an automatic guilty verdict.

The Ford Taurus turned on their police sirens, which were located inside of their vehicle. I said, **"Fuuu-cck**, I knew that was the feds." I felt relieved because I just stashed the gun and I no longer had anything illegal on me. Subsequently, the Ford Taurus pulled up on my vehicle. They rolled down the window and it was four, twenty something year old, white-boys, with that same buzz-light year haircut from the movie "Toy Story" that I had encounters with when I was an adolescent. This had to be De-Ja-Vu all over again. I couldn't believe it.

I remained calm because I didn't want to raise any suspicions as the "*ATF*" Agents steadily approached. I took inventory of what I had in the vehicle and realized that I still had the Baltimore dudes credit cards on me *"shoot,"* I said. I quickly devised an alibi, because I knew they were going to ask to search my vehicle. Cops always ask black people to step out of their vehicles so that they can search it, even when they aren't doing anything wrong. Heck, it could be for things as innocuous as a minor traffic stop and the cops are going to ask you if they can search your vehicle, and that's if they don't yank you out through the window by your arm first. Don't be a citizen on parole or probation? They are adamantly making you get out of your vehicle, no questions asked. Ain't no cop asking you politely to do shit if you're on community control! Consider yourself **Fuuu-cckkddt.** Knowing this, I figured I would tell the undercover agents that my classmates gave me a ride to campus and must have forgotten their credit cards in my vehicle, and I'd return it to them during the next class period. No sweat, right?

As the undercover, "*ATF*" agents approached the vehicle, I said, "Hey Marcus, listen up, don't say anything and remain calm, I have a plan. Sure, as the clouds are grey this bozo throws a monkey wrench directly into my plans and abruptly yells out, "I got a double-barrel shotgun and cocaine in this car!"

I responded, angrily, "SheeedN'Me, you ain't got no coca-hinya and guns in this car!" My face turned from a furious purple color to a bright plum red. I vexedly said, "What the hell are you doing in college with coke and a gun? Ain't no crackheads enrolled here dummy, unless you're using?"

Marcus replied, "It's my grandfather's shotgun, I stole it from his house when I was selected to attend Morgan State University. I don't trust these Baltimore dudes; they might try and blow my brains out my scalp given the opportunity." I looked to the right passenger seat and thought to myself this dude is from Largo, Maryland. A place where most people consider the suburbs. Prince George's County, Maryland is one of the richest counties in the United States. I 'thunk to myself, this guy must be paranoid if he thinks he needs to bring a shotgun to college with him because we're in East Baltimore. I mean damn, it is perilous, but if you feel like you need to carry a gun to walk back and forth to class everyday as a freshman in college then you really need to reconsider matriculating to another school. But that's how most *HBCU's in the inner-city of every urban section in America is. That's why it's never a black person's first choice when searching for colleges. It's usually their last resort. Sad but true. That's a paradox.*

I snapped out of my deep thought, and said, "You saw me trying to bust Doe boy, old, rusty ass .38caliber, why didn't you tell me that you had a shotgun? I could've used it to blow them dudes up from here to Baghdad."

Marcus said, "Exactly, that's why I didn't feel at liberty to disclose to you that I had it, I knew you would use it and I ain't trying to go to jail."

I hesitated, before replying, "SheeedN'Me, "How are you not trying to go to jail? Didn't you just say that you have cocaine, in my truck, foolio?"

Marcus replied, "Yes, but again, the cocaine is so I can sell it to pay for my college tuition, room and board."

Perplexed, I stated, "You were planning on paying your college tuition with drug money? That's ridiculous, but I won't be a hypocrite because I did the same thing. You can't throw stones when you live in a glass house." He replied, "Thanks for understanding."

The undercover *"ATF"* agent was now knocking on my driver's side window. I rolled the window down as he stated, *"License and Registration please!"*

I turned my head to the left and said, "License and registration, for what? Why are you pulling me over? To be defiant was not my intention, I was trying to buy time by asking questions, while conjuring in my head what my next move would be.

Before the agent could respond, I mashed he gas. Thus, a high-speed chase ensued. If you were a bystander that happened to witness me press on the gas pedal with overwhelming sheer force? You would've thought that I was running from a *melee*. My Nissan Pathfinder went from 0-60 miles per hour with alacrity, in just under ten seconds, which was arbitrarily fast for a truck that size. I told Marcus to put his seat belt on because we were about to go for a wild ride. I quickly turned the corner and drove towards West Baltimore, off North Avenue, so Marcus could get rid of the drugs and guns. I drove down Hillen road and they must've called back up because police squad cars swarmed down upon us from every direction, creating a barricade at the traffic light with their cars, as if that was going to preclude me from running. I stepped on the gas pedal until it touched the floor. I was going to run straight through them, without any contrition.

The squad cars retreated as I neared hitting them with my Nissan Pathfinder, I was determined to elude the "ATF" agents and the Baltimore police squad cars that were chasing me simultaneously and obviously drove vehicles that were much faster than mines, but desperate times call for desperate measure, so I gave it all I had. I told myself that I would not be taken to jail alive, they were going to have to kill me. I grew exasperated of jail at this point, I was over it. The only way they would apprehend, and house me inside a jail cell again was going to be in a pine box and I wasn't prepared for a funeral was my mind state. I drove around the circle in Druid Hill Park and the officers were still tailing me; as I pivoted the vehicle, they turned in hot pursuit. They were on my tail with precision. I couldn't shake em, although I did my best to.

I drove through a seedy looking neighborhood on Park Heights Avenue, between Slade Avenue and Park Village Court and yelled to

Marcus, "hurry, throw everything out the car, *nowwww*." I glanced in the rear-view mirror and noticed the neighborhood people that **were** on the sidewalk, jet into the street to pick up the guns and drugs. I felt a huge solace of *ree-liief* as I gasped for air so I wouldn't begin to hyperventilate and give myself an anxiety attack. The key to fleeing and eluding cops in a high-speed chase is to always remain poised and maintain control of the situation the best way that you can. However, Marcus didn't share the same sentiment. He began yelling, "Ahmed, we're going to die, they're going to kill us."

I looked over at Marcus, who was suddenly overcome with acute, severe anxiety. I noticed a wet puddle on his lap. I assumed he spilled a bottle of water on his jeans. I looked around and there was no bottle of water in the car. I realized, Marcus, pissed on himself, out of fear, he could no longer control his urethral sphincter. He urinated all over his pants and his shirt. Then he began crying hysterically. Actual tears, pouring out his eyes, like rain pouring from the sky. He even inadvertently threw his phone out the passenger-side window, so we had no sense of direction, whatsoever, he was so *shook, like a half-way crook*. I was once again incredulous, smitten, floored, as to the behavior of someone who personified a gangster persona and was turned out to be the complete opposite end of the spectrum. I knew nerds in college that were tough as nails, this dude was soft as cotton. He was becoming the epitome of a gangster rap-artist who sits in the studio all day long and rap about another person's life all the while disguising it as his own life. Like a magician, it was all an illusion. However, I still wanted to believe that it was the situation making him this way and not his actual character. Let me tell you something, when someone shows you who they are the first time, believe them. It will save you time from having to interact with them later in life, they become liabilities over assets. Just give people enough rope and eventually the ones who were not meant to be in your life will use that intangible rope to cut themselves off, and out of your life. It's actually one of the best lessons that you can learn in life. If you master the art of this method early on in life you learn to surround yourself with a fortress of stalwart men and women.

Aim High Push Hard

I'm not making light of his frantic state. He panicked and that's okay! What wasn't okay was he didn't display any bravery after being consumed by fear, which is a weak emotion. When faced with a trepidatious situation, your adrenal glands release catecholamines, which are your fight or flight response. You ultimately decide which one you would rather utilize given your level of bravery or cowardice. You either buckle up, lace your boot-straps and fight or you clam up like an oyster and get ready to take flight. I saw the exit sign for Interstate 95 South to Washington, D.C. But the gas tank meter showed empty before I could get on the highway, causing my Nissan Pathfinder to come to an abrupt halt.

I yelled to Marcus, "Get out the car and run as fast as you can, I'm out of gas, don't worry about me, save yourself, I was selfless. Get yourself to safety, we'll link back up later at school" I emphasized. Marcus did as I said and exited the vehicle with alacrity. The police squad car pulled up to the driver side of my vehicle and rammed the door, jamming it shut. I rolled down the driver's side window and jumped out, onto the hood of the patrol car, rolling off the hood of the patrol car and falling onto the street. I miraculously pulled myself together and got up and began running faster than Flash Gordon. The officer reversed the ca to create space, put the gear in drive and drove right into me, mowing me down like a lawn-mower. My legs gave out from the brutal impact, and I fell to the ground with muscle paralysis from the trauma I just sustained.

    A female officer handcuffed me and commenced to beating the black off my ass. Kicking me in my ribs and swiftly punching me in the face. I never got my ass beat that bad from a woman in my life. It was an ass whooping to remember, I felt like Rodney King. She then threw me in the back of the paddy wagon. Then got down to business and hauled my black ass off to Central booking detention center on East Madison Street, in Baltimore, Maryland. Damn, they caught me was all a brother was thinking. I gave them a hell of a run for their money, but they got my black ass hooked, lined and sinker. I was fumigating with rage. I'd rather died in the streets like a stuck-hog than go back to jail, again. The process is tedious as hell to endure. Not scary but boring, shameful, arduous, and I'd be remiss if I failed to mention the mental torment that going to jail takes on your family, fuck friends.

When you get arrested, your family is the only people that will *"try"* to be there for moral support. That's only if you *aren't* a jail bird, who doesn't mind being a frequent flyer to the bureau of prisons and your family has not lost all hope in you so they don't neglect you out of mindfulness that you may pull them down with you.

Financially, you're on your own. No one is going to keep spending all of their hard-earned money on you, (adolescent or adult) to repeatedly bail someone out of jail! It doesn't matter whether they are your family or not! People get exasperated with that kind of stuff, quick and in a hurry.

Chapter 8

Central Booking & Intake Center

I sat in a cell by myself for eight hours. Then a detective came and got me. He took me to a room with a table, two chairs and a bright fluorescent light in the middle. He let the light shine over my face, until it got scorching and small beads of sweat began to trickle down my forehead, before saying, "your friend Marcus snitched on you and confessed that the gun and drugs belonged to you."

"SheeedN'Me, I didn't have any drugs or guns. There is no way he could've told you something preposterous like that." I replied.

The detective retorted, "We have you on narcotics and weapons with ammunition charges. You will never see the light of day again." It suddenly dawned on me that police officers love saying that phrase to black men *"You will never see the light of day again.".* I thought back to when I was a child, and a police officer shared the same sentiment with me.

Police officers are just that, "overseers," who were bullied throughout their earlier years of school and then graduated high school and went to the police academy for a short duration of time to bully, harass, maim and murder black men. Let's be veracious, even cosmetologist must attend cosmetology school longer than police officers. So why do they yearn to be the judge, jury and executioner of every transgression so sedulously with draconian laws?

I was escorted back to my cell and the correctional officers brought Marcus into the cell with me. The first question he asked me was, "Did you tell the detective I had drugs and guns in the car? And they belonged to me?"

I responded, "they told me you said the same thing about me, something smells fishy here, I just can't put my nose to the scent. I don't think the detectives have a stalwart case and they're trying vehemently to get us to incriminate ourselves. Look, I insist we invoke our fifth amendment right to **shut the fuck up,** until we receive legal counsel." He agreed.

A few hours later, I went to see the commissioner for a bail review hearing. The first thing that she said was, "Wow, you have quite the lengthy criminal history sir, your bail will be set at *$75,000.00."* She proceeded, "You can either pay *10%* of *$75,000.00.00,* which is *$7,500.00* or you can remain incarcerated until your preliminary arraignment in 30 days, where your bail will either be increased or decreased." I began to realize that with every arrest, my bail was getting higher and higher. I finally realized that just like the healthcare industry; the judicial industry is also a business a seedy, exploitive, racist, bigotry business. You know what? Calling the "judicial system in America a business is dignifying it. They are a "gang" a "domestic terroristic gang." In my experience of dealing with law enforcement and the court system, it's always been about *"money." Sometimes I feel like you can buy your way out of trouble in America, contingent you have a surplus amount of cash laying around.*

I firmly stated, I have final exams tomorrow. I can't stay here for 30 days. I'll fail and have to repeat the semester." I called Fela. "I'm in jail for some bullshit and need you to call the bail-bondsmen and get me the heck up out of here." Fela said, "Say-less, I got you." I stayed in the central booking detention center for an additional 7 days before my bond cleared. During the interim, I learned to play chess, did sit-ups, push-ups and mostly scolded myself for making the same erroneous blunders repeatedly. I couldn't blame anyone but myself for my screw-ups in life.

The air conditioner in the jail was turned up, to maximum capacity. It felt like they wanted us to freeze to death in there and die from hypothermia. But, hey, Jail wasn't a hotel resort. I've been through enough trials and tribulations to understand that they make living conditions unbearable to deter you from wanting to come back. The irony is, once they put a "felony" conviction on your jacket? You mind as well cancel Christmas for the rest of your life, not just next year, because it's going to be in and out of prison like a cheap hostel for the rest of your natural life.

Once they have you on that felony radar, they know your choices of acquiring legal means of monetary funds are few and far in between so they keep one eye on you like the logo for the channel "CBS," 'cause they are more than aware that chances are you will be back to visit again sooner than later. Just look at the statistics for the African-American recidivism rate for the past fifty years and tell me what you extrapolate from your own research?

Meanwhile, we were sitting in jail at Central Booking in Baltimore, Maryland and Marcus was walking around with a blanket on shivering like a newborn baby with kernicterus. I yelled at him and asked him to take the blanket off.

I hollered, "You're around wolves and you're shivering? Wolves sense fear and they eat sheep." As soon as I said that the correctional officer yelled, "Ahmed, pack your bags, it's time to go, you've been bailed out."

Marcus said, "Ahmed, bail me out too." I turned back to him and said, "I got you." In the back of my mind, I was like, man fuck that bitch ass nigga. He acted like a pussy the entire time and has the nerve to ask me to bail him out? The gull and audacity of some negroes never ceases to amaze me. He showed me everything I needed to know and one thing I knew for certain was if the shoe was on the other foot, he wouldn't bail me out of jail. He would let me sit in there and rot like moldy bread. In life, one thing that you always have to do is look at the same scenario from the other person's perspective, i.e. what would they do if they were you? That thinking, and leading with your heart bullshit? Gon' get you late, ***every got-damn time.***

When I got out of the central booking detention center, the other inmates that were released with me, to my surmise, drove me back to Morgan State University. On the ride back, they said I left an indelible impression on them with how I carried myself during the short stint inside the jail. I made up my mind right then and there. This is it! no more trouble. I'm tired of living a criminal lifestyle, impressing convicts. What type of life is that? I keep taking trouble with me no matter where I go. I increased the level of the personal goals I set for myself to 21 credits per semester, all A's. No giving up no matter what, I came way too far in life to turn back now. I was much closer to where I was trying to go in life than I was to where I came from. The top was the destination. No road map, but I was determined to find my way and make it through like a compass. To be somebody in life that children could aspire to grow up and want to become. That was my goal.

Chapter 9

Final Mulligan

When I arrived back at Morgan State University, I scheduled appointments to meet with all my professors to plead with them to allow me to take the final exams that I missed. It was a long shot, but it was either that or back to the streets to sell drugs, 'cause working a 9-5? Was not on my mind at the time. That was not an option. My professors acquiescently complied and let me take the final exams, which were a piece of cake. I wish life was as easy as those final exams, with time to study and prepare for the difficulties that lay ahead. Instead of just wandering aimlessly and gambling on whether or not you make good decisions based on your past experiences. However, I digress. Against my better judgement and not wishing jail on my worst enemy. I bailed Marcus out of jail the next day in good faith that he would do something productive with his life. Boy, was I wrong.

When Marcus got out of jail. He told me that he was dropping out of college to go back to D.C. and sell crack full-time. His exact words were "College isn't for me." I was hurt and replied, "You do what you think is best for you and your current situation, but I'm going to medical school, and playing the long game." With that said, we parted ways. He went his way in life, and I went mines.

I enrolled in summer courses so I could finish college sooner. I excelled in all my classes and began studying for the medical college admissions test (MCAT). I also applied to Physician Assistant school simultaneously. In my mind, I figured what the heck? Why not try and kill two birds with one stone. Somehow, intrinsically, I believe, Marcus dropping out of school to go back to where he came from to sell crack, catapulted me in a way that I never expected it to. He probably doesn't know it but it had a profound impact on me. Because it was at that pivotal moment in my life, where I could have made a choice to go backwards, or to keep pushing forward, going against the grain, and grinding it out. No one ever said that life would be easy. The steps are always more difficult than climbing the elevator, yet it feels ***soooooo*** much ***bettttter*** when you sweat for it. ***Soooo muuuucccch beeeettteeeerrrr.*** My grade point average jumped from 3.501 to 3.768. I was accepted into the Physician Assistant program at the University of Maryland Eastern Shore (UMES). I was ecstatic.

I rescinded my Medical School application and graduated with a degree in Pre-Med Biology with honors. I ruminated over my options and decided it would prove prudent to pursue medical school later, my paper was running low after all those fines, bails, courts and lawyer fees. In Hindsight? Had it not been for my financial shortcomings, which I attribute to my mischievous behavior. I would have gone to medical school, unequivocally, no doubt. But life does what life does, and that is keep on lifing, so I chose to go with the flow and adhered to the program.

I skipped the Morgan State University graduation ceremony because I didn't want to walk across the stage and feel like I completed or accomplished anything yet. Mrs. Kilani was pissed but the mission that

I set out for myself was not complete, and this was the tactic that I thought I needed to utilize in order to motivate me to keep on climbing the ladder of success. I wanted to wear that white coat. I wanted to order and interpret diagnostic labs. Make troubling diagnosis, intricate treatment plans and prescribe the best medications for my patients to bring them back to normal baseline and optimal health. I wanted to ultimately give good health back to the same community that tried adamantly to take my life. It was my way of coping with my own mental trauma. Giving light to darkness heals me and giving love to hate soothes my once tortured soul from the dark abyss of the ghetto slums from where I dwelled.

Upon matriculating at the University of Maryland Eastern Shore, I noticed that there were Thirty-one students in my class. That seemed like a lot to me, considering the previous year they had less than 20 students in the graduating class. The age range was from 21 years old to 56 years old. On the first day of class, the brilliant Dr. Allen Tustin, who graduated from Vanderbilt University's Medical Program. Began asking questions that seemed simple to everyone else, yet they were bewildering to me. The first question he asked was, "Who can tell me what 'CO2' is?" Me, being the overzealous student, raised my hands up high and answered, "That is the cartridge that we used to insert into our B.B. guns when we played cops and robbers as children. The entire class laughed, which infuriated me, because I wasn't trying to be comedic. That was my definition of carbon dioxide at that time. I did not know any better but would soon learn that when you know better you do better.

Dr. Tustin replied, "That is incorrect, 'CO2' also known as carbon dioxide is the air that we expel out of our lungs, after we breathe in oxygen, which is carried by hemoglobin through the blood and exchanged for carbon dioxide in the alveoli, located in the bronchial tree of your lungs."

The next question Dr. Tustin asked was, "Class, who can tell me how many chambers the heart has?" I was salivating at the chance to redeem myself. I anxiously raised my hand and replied, "That's a trick question Dr. Tustin, the heart is an organ, composed of muscle fibers, it doesn't have any chambers." Once again, the entire class laughed at my ignorance, which vexed me even more than the previous question. If this were the game-show jeopardy, the host "Alex Trebek" would have thrown me off the show for answering questions blatantly, arrogantly and incorrectly. I felt ashamed and humiliated by my own ignorance.

Dr. Tustin stated, "What is your name young man?" I replied, Ahmed Gbadamosi Sir." Dr. Tustin retorted, "Well Ahmed, I don't know if you're joking or not? But it appears to me as though you don't have a clue about medicine or how the human body works. Physician Assistant school is like Medical School. The only distinct but subtle difference is, instead of attending four years of Medical School. Physician Assistant School is crammed into two years, so you need to decide today whether medicine is the career you would like to choose? Because, I'll be honest with you Ahmed, there are a million other careers that pay a lot more than medicine. You will also get more sleep than becoming a doctor. Medicine is an altruistic career; everyone can't do it. You either have what it takes to succeed, or you don't. And I'll be veracious with you

Ahmed, I don't think that you have what it takes based on the erroneous answers that you just gave. A feeling of dismay came over me after hearing those words roll off his tongue. I didn't like that feeling. I never wanted to feel it again. I made a mental mote that something had to change with my myopic knowledge base of medicine at the time, I was still considered a rook, wet hind the ol'ear.

Dr. Tustin then began asking the class, "How many of you all have had any medical experience prior to attending this school?" More than 95% of the class raised their hand. Some of the students said that they were paramedics, nurses, respiratory therapist, emergency medical technicians, pharmacists, army medical corps, certified nursing assistants, and medical assistants.

I thought to myself "Got-damn, I'm out of my league here, these muthafuckas smart as fuck, but I ain't going back to the hood to stand on that corner, pumping crack and busting guns at the opposition." Every time that I felt like quitting that was the chant that I would say to myself. It would *al-waaaays* rile me back up and get me in a good mood.

Aim High Push Hard

I went to Barnes and Nobles bookstore and bought every book they had in the medical aisle. I called my cell phone company and disconnected my phone services. I went home and took one look at my television, I unplugged it, picked it up, carried it outside and threw it in the dumpster. It was a distraction that had no use to me anymore. I perspicaciously understood the notion that if I wanted to truly become successful, reaching the heights I set for myself, I would have to cut off all communication with the outside world, they were all distractions to me at that point in my life. I had to be disciplined. That meant no girlfriend, no junk food, no parties, no sporting events, no camping trips, no fishing, no boating, no chilling, no hanging, no nothing, straight work, all day and all night.

The next day I awoke and went to Walmart to buy a weber charcoal grill. I then went to Costco to purchase a membership card. I bought a months' worth of poultry and fish. I also bought a deep freezer that was on sale to store all the poultry and fish inside.

My rationale was that I would grill a weeks' worth of food every Sunday morning. This in turn would increase my study time during the week because I would not have to waste precious time cooking breakfast, lunch and dinner, every night, when I could be studying.

I felt as though I was running a marathon race. Except, I was in last place. I understood that If I wanted to win this marathon, I would have to work harder, faster and more diligently than everyone else in my class. I did 100 push-ups every morning followed by 100 sit-ups. At night, after my last class, I ran 3 miles daily to stimulate the release of endorphins. I understood a huge part of my success depended on my dopamine and serotonin levels to be at an all-time high. I needed to be revved up. **Caffeinated-up and motivated-up!** The bottom line is if you want it, then you have to go out and get it. You don't have to be the best. You just have to do your best. That's all anyone can ask of you. Keep in mind, no one is going to give a thing to you. You have to scratch, claw and fight for every penny.

Chapter 10

Metamorphosis

My classes were Monday through Friday. Classes began at 7am prompt, and ended at 9pm, roughly. With various reprieves in between. The first year of Physician Assistant school epitomized medical boot-camp. It certainly was rigorous and challenging but I felt confident in my preparation.

The first class of the day was Anatomy and Physiology, the professors separated the classes so that the subject matter wouldn't be so difficult to comprehend. However, Physiology was arduous as heck, to say the least. It was comprised of learning about the human body from the molecular level. Learning about "ATP" Adenosine Triphosphate, which is a molecule that carries energy within cells. It's the main energy currency of the cell. In laymen terms, it is the powerhouse of the cell. Nothing works without Adenosine Triphosphate.

I also learned about the nucleus, which is the information center of the cell and is surrounded by a nuclear membrane. Humans' "DNA" (Deoxyribonucleic Acid) is stored inside the nucleus. Your genetic make-up and your identity are stored inside of the nucleus cell.

I learned about neutrophils, which serve as an essential part of the innate immune system. In layman's term, Neutrophils are like soldiers during war, they help you fight the battle by warding off bacterial infections. We then learned about macrophages, which are also important cells of the immune system, that are formed in response to an infection or accumulating damaged or dead cells. In layman's term, macrophages are identical to ballistic missiles during war. They recognize the enemy, i.e., infection, then they engulf and destroy the target cells. I call macrophages, "the little rocket men of the immune system*." Like Donald Trump refers to North Korean President, Kim Jong-Un aka "little*

rocket man." Furthermore, macrophages destroy invading microorganisms through a process called *phagocytosis.*

Phagocytosis, which means, simply "to eat" are white blood cells. They are a vital part of the immune system, after the neutrophils and macrophages fight the war, leaving enemies, i.e., bacteria lying dead on the battlefield. Henceforth, *phagocytosis* is the process of eating everything up, which aids in protecting the body.

The next topic of discussion was lymphocytes, which are blood cells that are also an integral part of the immune system. I learned that there are two types of *lymphocytes. B cells and T cells,* which derive from the thymus gland when we were children. The *B cells* produce antibodies that are used to attack invading bacteria, viruses and toxins. The *T cells* protect people from getting infected by destroying cancerous and infected cells.

Now, let's discuss anatomy, "Anatomy Lab" to be specific. Anatomy lab was one of the best classes that I'd ever taken in my entire life. It was a class full of *dead bodies*, basically, cadavers, which were human beings, whose last wishes before their demise was to donate their bodies to medical schools for research science. The bodies were usually freshly preserved so you could smell the embalming fluid permeating from their skin. I quickly began to dissect the bodies. I approached the course with an alacrity of yearning to know what the human body looked like internally. I put a mask on the faces of the cadavers so that it could distort my mind from thinking about the life of the person that I was cutting on. Other students were not as unbridled as I was. Some students got dizzy and fainted upon dissection of the cadavers, I'm talking full blown syncopal episode! Passed out, flatlined, face first on the floor. Other students vomited and could not continue with the course, so they conceded and dropped out of PA school all together, which was sorely disappointing, but I was able to understand that it is better to walk away with dignity instead of wasting time doing something that you dislike. Sometimes change is better. Perhaps, that may have been the best decision for my classmates. Who knows? Maybe the students went on to find their true interest in life and pursued other subjects and careers that they were passionate about.

In my personal belief, anatomy class can quickly help you decide whether medicine is a **passion** or just a field that you would like to pursue for **financial gain.** Remember what I said earlier about Dr. Tustin saying, "There were easier professions, where you can make more money than being a *Physician Assistant/Medical Doctor?*" Well, this class separated the boys from the men and the girls from the women. The bravery and gusto possessed inside of your soul had to either be innately born inside you or it just wasn't. **Point blank period!** *I mean that with no contrition.*

I became official like a referee with a whistle. I was jubilant to learn about what arteries supplied specific organs. What veins drained each organ, and what nerves innervated each muscle. I felt like an 11-year-old kid going to Disneyworld for the first time. I was pumped and ready to learn. I thought to myself, "Oh yeah, this class is going to be an easy A+ for me." The only discrepancy I had was that there were not enough cadavers for all of us students to dissect each body on our own. Predominantly because the Physician Assistant students had to share the Anatomy lab room with the Physical Therapy students.

Since anatomy was more of an integral component of physical therapy. They always got first dibs on all the "Dead-Bodies." There would be 16 students, at any given time, poking and cutting off the skin around the forehead to pull the skin off the face. Using a power drill to crack the skull open to explore the four areas of the brain. Slicing the penis open to view the corpus cavernosum or splitting the vagina down the middle to explore the uterus, ovaries and the rest of the female reproductive system that gives rise to a newborn baby. It truly was an inspirational moment for me. However, the physical therapy students were hovered all around the few *dead bodies* that were available inside the frigid cold anatomy lab room. I decided to leave the class and utilize that time to study for my physiology exams. I said to myself, "I will come back inside here on Friday and Saturday night, that way, most of the students will likely be out partying. The other students will be spending precious time with their children or just at home relaxing watching a movie to ease their mind from all the rigorous studying during the weekdays."

I had a vehement disdain for the rigmarole way of doing things. Friday night came, and I went for a three-mile brisk jog to ease the tension and to get my mind right. Then headed to anatomy lab at 12:00 am. Just as I thought, there was no one there except myself and the cadavers. I had the lab all to myself. I exclaimed, **"Yes, let's work."**

I unzipped the first body-bag, and the face was not covered so my reflexes caused me to become startled as I jumped back in terror. In anatomy lab, it was customary to cover the faces with a bag or wash cloth whenever students finish off with his or her dissection. It wasn't enforced by the professors, but it was the "consideration" that mattered amongst the students.

At any rate, me having developed tough-skin from the hood, I re-grouped and got myself back together. As I began anatomizing the chest cavity to explore the heart and lungs. I couldn't help but marvel at all the other cadavers zipped up in body bags and I proceeded to say out loud "I absolutely, unequivocally, *could not* become a mortician, there is no way I can sit around dead people all day cutting them open. Dissecting them is one thing but polishing faces, putting puddy on wounds and the other mundane logistics of being an actual mortician is not for me."

I pressed on, as I made a surgical incision into the thoracic area of the cadaver in front of me laying on the table, when suddenly, the other body bags jumped up. I said, *"What the heck is that?* I answered myself incredulously to ease the mental tension. Rigor mortis setting in?" I hastily proceeded, then another body jumped up and another and another. I said, *"Mehnn, forget this,* they're coming back alive, the cadavers aren't dead, they are ghost coming back to haunt me. I'm getting the hell up out of here." I scurried my scary behind back to my apartment quicker than Flash Gordon. I went to my room, jumped in the bed and pulled the covers over my head and fell fast asleep.

The next morning, I woke up and decided to face my fears, I went right back into that "Anatomy lab room". There were some upper-classroom physical therapy students inside the lab room, so I decided to tell them about my experience from the previous night and they began laughing their butts off. I looked at them with scorn and contempt as I asked, "Why are you all laughing at me? It's not funny, I was terrified out of my mind."

One of the Physical Therapy upper-class students asked, "Ahmed have you noticed how cold it is inside here?

I replied, "Yes, it's freezing in here at all times.

The upper-class student stated, "Look up at the vents, do you notice how hard the air is blowing out of them?"

I said, "Yes, I do. What's your point?"

The physical therapy student replied, "The force from the air blowing through the vent blows the body-bags left and right so that's probably what you were hearing, *"Air blowing dead body bags"*.

Aim High Push Hard

I remained firm on my stance, that I believe I saw the cadaver bodies bumping and jumping in and out of those bags. I was almost certain that it was surely not just air moving those cadaver body bags.

The upper-class man took me around each individual body, zipped the body-bag and poked and probed them. He said, "Ahmed, every cadaver in here is as good as *"Dead"*. That was just your mind playing tricks on you.

I was ashamed. I felt like a *"cowardice goofball"*. Whether air was blowing through the vents moving the body-bags or rigor mortis setting into the cadavers? I never went back to anatomy lab at night by myself anymore. I decided to tough it out and attend anatomy lab during the weekdays with the other students from my class. I was spooked like Casper the unfriendly ghost, case closed!

Chapter 11

Residency #1

When I began rotations in my second year of PA school, I felt like I finally found peace and freedom. I no longer had to sit in class for an inordinate number of hours listening to professors belabor me about medicine. I could begin applying everything I learned into real world practical scenarios.

My initial residency was OB-GYN. I wanted to get it out of the way because I had a weak stomach for probing around the genital areas of men, women, boys and girls. Human genitalia is not my forte. It was part of the job, and my preceptor didn't make it any easier for me.

His name was Dr. Illupeju. He owned his practice on New Hampshire Avenue in Washington D.C.

He lived in the same building he practiced in. That's how I knew he was Nigerian and frugal, that's typical Naija behavior, i.e., "live where they work in order to reduce their expenses." Cheapskates! Let's just call a spade a spade on this one guys. That is my culture and I know them through and through. *Nigerians are certified cappers!* Not all of them, but most of them are "flaw" as hell. Pretentious as fuck. Ever since they watched the movie called, *"Coming to America,"* they all think that they are *Hakeem.* Eddie Murphy's character. They lure you in with frivolous banter about how they are kings in their countries back home, that shit is all CAP.   He lived upstairs and used the basement to do pelvic exams and consultations on women with genitourinary diseases. Mainly, endometriosis, fibroids, polycystic ovarian disease, etc... He didn't deliver babies because he stated, "The malpractice insurance is just too high." But I knew that he was just too cheap to pay for it.

At any rate this man scolded me routinely. I assumed it was tough love because we were both from Nigeria and ironically, we were both from the same Yoruba tribe. He would come downstairs with his cup of coffee and dip his slice of wonder bread inside of it and state, loudly "the attending is here." Be mindful the start time was 8:00am Mon-Friday for thirty days and he would show up blissfully late at 9:30am. I felt that he was narcissistic, arrogant and self-entitled, but I kept my comments to myself.

The first patient he gave me was an 80-year-old woman who he suggested "would be good practice." That was a bold face lie because he never gave me any of the young patients, he just didn't want to do pelvic exams on the older patients himself. He gave me a creepy vibe but like I said I needed to pass this residency in order to move on to the next residency.

I walked into the exam room with a chaperone, who happened to be a certified nursing assistant, (and said to myself, "thank God he can afford one of those, this guy is cheap." The nurse prepped the patient who was now laying on the bed with each leg in stirrups.

Dr. Illupeju asked me to tell the patient to "lift her but off the table and scoot up." Which, I did, but what he did next, I was not prepared for. He shined a bright lamp over my head as he stood behind me and pushed my face into the lady's vagina. He said "You must get inside there if you want to do a two-finger bimanual exam. It was gross and I began to sweat profusely because the lady started moaning like she was being sexually pleasured. I began feeling nauseous, and the smell protruding from between her legs was horrific.

I could not decipher if it were a lack of proper hygiene from old age? or she just didn't wash? Or decayed flesh, however, it was horrible. Rancid smell. Albeit I kept my composure and after the bimanual exam I had to do the pelvic exam to rule out cervical dysplasia, again he palmed the back of my head, and I was face to face with this 80yr/old woman's vagina. I quickly asked the nurse for the speculum. I then asked the patient to take a deep inhalation as I inserted the speculum. I asked the nurse for the culture swab and rubbed the cervix, then quickly gave it back to the nurse so she could send the sample to quest diagnostics for testing. I said to the patient, "This concludes the exam, Ma'am. She replied, "I like you; it was quick and painless, I need to go outside and smoke a cigarette." Dr. Illupeju began laughing at my disdain as I ran outside the clinic and into the alley to avoid being seen vomiting. I felt like I had just been through hazing. Similar to the way fraternities haze the new pledges, who are coming on-board at collegiate institutions, I was infuriated at Dr. Illupeju for what transpired. I got myself together and walked back into the medical room, with my chin up, and my chest out as if the events that occurred earlier didn't bother me.

The first thing Dr. Illupeju said was, "Ahmed, I need you to go back into the patients' room, take the speculum and put it in hot water so that we can use it for the next patient." I replied, "That is unsanitary, PA school taught us to throw away speculums and use brand-new unopened packs for each patient so as to not re-introduce infection to the patient.   Furthermore, that is unethical and if the patients were aware that we were reusing speculums they would be upset and file a medical malpractice claim." He looked at me with indignation in his eyes, and said, "This isn't school, this is my private practice, do you know how much each speculum cost me? These expenses are coming out of my pocket, you are my PA student, so you do what I tell you to do." I acquiescently complied and just shook my head, as I mumbled under my breath, "This African Bambaataa looking face muthafuckah here thinks he is *Hakeem* off of *"Coming to America"* for real, what's up with this dude? I felt that negative frequency between us off the top. I knew we would not gel well. As I write this novel, growing up in America and having the privilege to travel back and forth to Nigeria and west Africa. I've never once in my life meshed well with Nigerian men or women. It's always been a challenging experience in my lifetime.

I then went to the bathroom to wash my hands. As I came out of the washroom, I threw the napkin that I used to dry my hands into the trash bin. Dr. Illupeju saw that and became irate. His face fill with disconcertment, as He said, infuriated, "Do you know how much I pay for napkins? I replied, "No, I don't, but honestly, I was apathetic as to the cost. I was doing my job as a student medical practitioner. He then stated sarcastically, "Too much for you to throw away a napkin after one use, you take that napkin out of the trash can and use it at least two to three times before discarding it." I mumbled under my breath, "Are you serious?" He replied, "What did you say?" I responded hesitantly, "Nothing sir, and picked the napkin back out of the trash can and put it back into the pockets of my lab coat. I was one week through my OB-GYN residency and dreaded the fact that I had to be there for another three weeks. But as Sigmund Freud once said, "One day in retrospect the years of struggle will strike you as the most beautiful."

    I just couldn't compose myself that night when I went home to try to relax and get some rest for the evening. Dr. Illupeju was on my mind all night. Thoughts were just brimming in my brain; why is this man treating me this way? Why is he so cheap? Does he hate me? Does it have something to do with some Nigerian cultural beliefs of hazing that I'm unaware of? Is he projecting his fears onto me."

Aim High Push Hard

Whatever it was, I had to ascertain the truth for myself, it was that important to me. While lying in bed I made a vow to have a one-on-one discussion with Dr. Illupeju the next morning. Whether he was my Preceptor or not, I'm a man, my word and self-respect are all I possess in this cold world, I cogitated to myself. The greatest truths in life are usually the most unpleasant to hear but I needed to hear the truth. I couldn't live on a lie. But I could stand on the truth and accept it. Regardless of how hurtful or ugly the truth was to hear.

The next morning, I awoke for residency and made sure to stop at Panera bread and grab a blueberry bagel lightly toasted with cream cheese and a cup of warm green tea to ensure my energy would be right before I walked into the office. I made certain to grab extra napkins from Panera bread and stuffed each pocket of my lab coat with them. I was done with that recycling napkins crap. I just wasn't in the mood to sip the tea for that fever *chilllleeee'd.*

As I drove to work munching on my blueberry lightly toasted, cream cheese bagel. I kept telling myself no matter what happens today, don't let them see me sweat, keep my cool and remember that good things usually happen, bad things sometimes happen.

I reached Dr. Illupeju's office at 8:00am prompt. I went over the enumerated list of patients and the diseases that I would have to treat for the day. Dr. Illupeju wasn't there yet so I opened my epocrates medical drug book and researched side-effects and dosages of medications that I would need to ascertain and commit to memory just in case patients had questions about their ailments. I implored myself to be prepared.

Just as I began scrutinizing Gonadotropin-releasing hormone agonists like Lupron; Which, works by blocking the production of estrogen and progesterone, by putting you into a temporary menopause-like state. I learned that Lupron was a drug that could improve fibroid symptoms. However, it causes unpleasant menopausal symptoms such as hot flashes. I figured If I could alleviate the stress from my mid-aged female patients by telling them, "I found a drug that precludes menstrual periods and shrinks fibroids so that surgery can become a last resort option for the patient, they would be ecstatic to hear the good news." Basically, anything I could do to help alleviate a woman's abdominal pain and heavy, painful, vaginal bleeding without invasive surgery is what I was willing to do.

Dr. Illupeju was a pro surgery type of surgeon, who would recommend surgery as soon as possible to cut a problematic lesion out of a woman's uterus. That's how he made his money, and that's how he paid his bills, so I had to respect it. I had no choice but to. However, I'm the type of medical practitioner that puts himself in another person's shoes prior to making a life altering decision and albeit, I don't know what it's like to be a woman living with painful fibroids that are the size of golf balls on her uterus. I'm certain that I wouldn't want anyone cutting into my testicles as a first resort option if there's a medication that could help preclude it. I'd elect to try the medication first. I felt that others would have similar sentiments if they were aware of *all* their options in totality. Furthermore, I understood there were different variables-such as how sick a patient is? The patients' age? Whether the patient has any pending co-morbidity diseases that coincides with the risks of surgery? There are always several careful questions to answer and variables to consider prior to deciding on slicing someone open in an operating room. I'm adamant about being meticulous when making such an arduous decision because of the *way I was sliced open by that resident as a kid*, although the resident had good intentions and saved my life. I sincerely believe she could've used better tact and skill in how she proceeded *to slice me open*. Sometimes it's not about what you do but how you do it that matters the most. As I became absorbed in profound thought, Dr. Illupeju walks in at 9:30am, blissfully late as per usual with not a care in the world about the student's time, with his cup of coffee in hand, along with bread to dip inside his coffee, his "breakfast of champions."

He blurts out, "The attending is here, Ahmed, are you prepared to present the first patient?" I replied, "yes sir, however, can I speak to you briefly in your office about a personal matter that is bothering me?" He replied snarky, bothering you? what could possibly be bothering you at this stage in your life, you are too young to know suffering, me, I'm a Naija man, the worst that life has to offer a human being in America, is equivalent to the best that life has to offer a human being where I come from." We walked into his office, and I shut the door behind me as he took a seat behind his cluttered desk.

I replied, "Do you hate me sir?"

He said, "Hate you? Why would I hate you?"

I said, "for starters the way you palmed the back of my head and roughly shoved it closely to the patient's vagina yesterday while shining that bright lamp over my head made me nauseous."

I didn't want him to know that I went outside to vomit after the pelvic exam procedure yesterday. I didn't want him to think I was a *wimp*. My pride and ego combined wouldn't allow me to tell him the entire truth. Something I learned to let go of as I matured with age.

He stated, "Ahmed, If I hated you, I wouldn't be so hard on you. I've seen you reading before each patient arrives and after each patient leaves, constantly staying abreast with information and innovative ways to treat patients. Ahmed, I know that you are a sedulous student, but I want you to work as diligently as humanly possible to reach your full potential. Nobody's too good and nobody's good enough but we're from Nigeria, which means that we must work ten times as hard and be ten times as good to make it in this world.

I was speechless, that is not the response I expected but fate loves to astonish us with irony and maybe I was over-thinking things, which caused me to overreact. I sat in my chair and thought to myself, "wow, some people show love in different ways and since I never had a personal relationship with my own father, I never experienced this type of love before, or any type of love for that matter. I grew a newfound respect for Dr. Illupeju that day.

Subsequently, the next three weeks went smooth as margarine-butter. I assisted on a patient with widespread endometriosis, who presented to clinic weeks prior to procedure, and described, dysmenorrhea (menstrual pain that was far worse than usual as her primary symptom), along with dyspareunia (pain with intercourse), dyschezia (pain with bowel movements), and menorrhagia (heavy menstrual bleeding)

Dr. Illupeju made sure to take his time during this surgery and the other surgeons teased him, saying things like, "He holds up the surgical room for inordinately long periods of time, sometimes for 10 hours at a time for a surgery that could be performed in 3 to 5 hours. Dr. Illupeju was aware that the other surgeons despised him and talked behind his back, but he didn't let it bother him, he ignored them. His theory was if it's one thing you can depend on people being? *it's people, and everyone has the right to their own opinion.* He exhorted me to always follow my intuition and take my time during invasive surgical procedures because it can mean the difference between life or death.

Chapter 12

Residency#2

My next residency was emergency medicine. I knew that I would love the emergency room before I stepped foot inside of one. I grew up watching every episode of "ER," an American medical drama television series created by novelist and physician Michael Crichton that aired on NBC from September 19, 1994, to April 2, 2009. The show is the second longest-running primetime medical drama behind *Grey's Anatomy*, and the sixth longest medical drama across the globe.

I knew I would grow up to be a doctor like George Clooney, Anthony Edwards, Noah Wyle, Eriq La Salle and Mekhi Phifer. The characters they played resonated with me profoundly. I loved the way they would always be on their toes; each Doctor's adrenaline rushing whenever there was a mass casualty incident. A mass casualty incident

(MCI) is defined as "an event that overwhelms the local healthcare system, where the number of casualties exceeds the local resources and capabilities in a short period of time.

Day number one in the Emergency room was all gas no breaks. Working in a level-1 trauma center felt supernatural. I treated everything from gunshot wounds, sharp object penetrations, fractured bones, tension pneumothorax, pulmonary embolism, pericardial tamponades, cardiac arrest (heart attack), to cerebrovascular accidents and transient ischemic attacks (stroke/mini-stroke).

I was permitted to suture lacerations from knife penetrations, which resonated with me profoundly because I was also stabbed in my chest, arm, and back as a juvenile. The doctor that sutured my wounds sped through it and left me with hideous scars that were displeasing and made me feel unattractive, however, the painful scars built and shaped my character to be relentless in my pursuit of medicine.

Aim High Push Hard

When my juvenile patients were presented to the emergency room with gunshot wounds with a mental component attached behind it; I noticed that I empathized with these patients more than the average physician because I understood what they were going through from personal experiences. Henceforth, my work was not complete after I brought the patient back to normal baseline.

I personally assured to link them with a social support system, a therapy group, a counseling session where they could speak to people with similar experiences, so they don't wind up repressing their feelings of discontentment, which later in life leads to depression and social isolation. Thus, ruining opportunities they may have acquired before receiving an opportunity to attain them. That's the quickest way to crash and burn for a black man. Unfortunately, that previous statement is ubiquitous amongst black men residing in urban areas. And they wonder why it's hard being black.

I believed it was my obligation because I also was a product of their environment, a lawless land where its kill or be killed. Where you're taught to meet aggression with aggression. You take one of mine. I take two of yours and the cycle reverberates, generation after generation. After I took a bullet to my right atrium as a child, it was the last time I felt truly safe. Whoever shot me on my birthday stole from me a sense of security. That is what violation does; it wrenches away one's God-given freedom to exhale, to feel relaxed and unguarded in this world.

    I deferred from the doctors and nurses in the emergency room by the personal experiences I shared with my patients, experiences they related to. what I shared similar, personal experiences with my patients, where I felt like my God given right to breath and walk the streets innocuously was taken away. When someone violates you, it does not simply haunt and aggrieve you; it alters the very shape of your soul. You feel as though your heart has been sliced wide-open, you tend to haphazardly hurl rocks in every direction. You want someone, anyone, to ache and bleed as badly as you have.

    I was confounded by the amount of senseless gunshot wounds that came into the emergency room on an hourly basis. Sadly prescient, I wasn't oblivious to the fact that these kids would have no choice but to return to the same environment where our spirits fail to dull the traumatic, when our physical is still surrounded by the spirits that caused the traumatic incident.

I would always leave each juvenile and adult patient who survived a gunshot or sharp object penetration wound with words of divinity instilled in me through God's vessel. I told them that there's a path in this life with your name on it. What God means for you to have, no one can take away from you. It's already yours. Our mission, as God's children is to surrender to what he has ordained—and to freely let all else just pass us by.

Furthermore, I knew deep down in my heart that just walking through this life as a black person, and actually surviving that, was and still is an ovation worthy of performance. But hey, if you can be black and live in this world, you can be anything you want to be. That is why it's vital to know your history. When you know your history, you know your value. You know the price that has been paid for you to be here.

During my next three weeks, I had a 15yr/old patient that came in with seventeen stab wounds all over his face. Which was covered in blood. He had a red bandanna tied around his head, which indicated to me that he was affiliated with the "bloods" a gang that originated in Los Angelas, California. He presented to the emergency room with his grandmother, and she was sobbing hysterically.

I began asking the pertinent questions, "What happened to you?" "Who did this to you?" "Can you raise your eyebrows?" Then I proceeded, "Can you smile, frown and you wrinkle your forehead?" "Do you feel any numbness on your face?" To ensure that he had no compromise of the facial nerve. The facial nerve controls the muscles that help you smile, frown, wrinkle your nose, and raise your eyebrows and forehead. The facial nerve is known as the seventh cranial nerve, which performs motor and sensory function.

If I could not appreciate that these nerves were not compromised by having the patient perform these sensory and motor functions, although he was under immense pain and duress. I would have to send him up to the operating room for a surgical procedure. Before the young man could utter a word, his grandmother interjected; "His father is in prison and his mom is a prostitute addicted to heroin, I took legal guardianship of him at four-years old, but I just can't handle him on my own, he doesn't listen to anything I say, and this is not the first time he was stabbed."

However, the young man followed my command and performed the task I asked of him by moving all the muscles in his face and there was no trigeminal nerve dysfunction, upon physical exam. The trigeminal nerve (the fifth cranial nerve, or simply CN V) is a nerve responsible for sensation in the face and motor functions such as biting and chewing: it is the most complex of the cranial nerves. All I could think to myself was thank you God, because I did not want this young boy to have to undergo a facial reconstruction in the operating room at the tender age of fifteen. Along with the facial scar from the reconstruction surgery that would leave an indelible mental scar that he would never be able to get rid of. The agony would be too much to bear. I didn't want to exacerbate his trauma. To my amazement the young boy was cool, calm and collected, which perplexed me because being stabbed twice before the age of sixteen is not normal. But, in the African American community; unfortunately, physical trauma is common, recurrent, and habitual. We understand it because we see it on a day-to-day basis. Getting shot or stabbed before your sixteenth birthday is like receiving a black eye from a fight in the hood. We used to call it the neighborhood, but the repetitious violence ran all the neighbors away, so we coined it "the hood."

I then proceeded to grab some Kleenex tissue and wiped the tears from his grandmother's exhausted face and asked if she could step into the waiting room while I worked to suture the 17 lacerations on this young boy's face. I commenced treating the facial lacerations with initial pain control, utilizing topical "LET" Lidocaine, epinephrine, tetracaine) rather than infiltrative anesthesia. I asked the nurse to get me the finest 6-0, vicryl sutures that we had to achieve optimal cosmetic results, I knew this boy would be facially disfigured for life and I wanted to perform a great job in order to minimize the scarring as he aged. I practiced suturing in school on pig arms and watched a ton of you tube videos on how to suture limbs, appendages, faces and arms effectively. However, this was my first time suturing a human being. I seized the opportunity; however, I was cautious as I didn't want to make a mistake.

This was my opportunity to project my own self-awareness that I was as good as I thought I was. I didn't call my preceptor for guidance or assistance. I wanted to do this on my own. It feels better when you sweat for it. This was my time to shine. I felt like I was at a championship game, and I was the underdog. That's the excitement, the stimulation of the sympathetic nervous system, the adrenaline that you feel when met with this type of high-acuity, facial injury. The trauma, the blood, the fatty-adipose tissue. To suture multiple lacerations effectively on a patient's face is not an art, but a skill. You can quote me on that.

I was nervous but confident in my ability to prove to myself, and to my preceptor, that I didn't choose medicine as a career. Medicine chose me! With that thought in mind, I put on surgical gloves, sterilized the field and got to work. I irrigated the patient's face with fresh saline and cleansed the lacerations with antiseptic betadine. I palpated the wounds lightly and asked, "if he could feel any pain?" He replied, "No, just pressure." This young man was tough. Throughout the entire procedure he did not shed a tear. I was taken aback by his bravery. He showed signs of strength and confidence.

Paradoxically, you can teach a child a new skill, whether bowling or how to play pool to precision but you can't instill in him or her the confidence, bravery, strength and courage it takes for one to endure painful hardships, time and time again. It's daunting and sadly, it never gets any easier. Problems are a part of life, you become stronger at pulling from thoughts of choices you made from previous existential experiences, and you make different decisions. Thereby, dealing with the problem head-on and choosing the solution that has the least negative impact on our lives. I don't believe we possess the omnipotence to make the right decisions every time we're met with a trepidatious situation, but we can choose the least wrong one.

Upon suturing the patient's face, he was reticent, but as the procedure progressed, he began to express himself and uttered,

"Man, I knew I should've just let the crips have that chain."

"What chain?" I questioned.

He replied, "My big blood chain with the diamonds encrusted around it, I had to get jumped in on the set to get that chain and told myself I would die before ever letting someone snatch my chain off my neck."

I was bewildered, then said fiercely, "So you mean to tell me that you risk being stabbed in your face, 17 times over a chain?"

He then stated, "You're a doctor, you don't know about gang life and how valuable that chain is, it's more than a chain, it's the camaraderie the chain brings, I love the hood and my bloods more than life itself."

I shook my head in dismay and replied, "Young man, you haven't begun your life yet, you're still practically a baby and are ready to throw your life away over a chain? Listen to yourself."

He persisted, "I'll die for the bros and that's on gang."

It saddened me profoundly to hear this young man speak this way and I became disgruntled as I pushed the surgical suture tray to the side, and said, "now, normally I wouldn't do this because it's unethical, but you seem like the type of teenager who believes in seeing, rather than hearing as I lifted up my shirt to show him my wounds." The patient was astounded by the sight of my healed scars. It appeared to take his breath away as he looked on amazed and confounded.

He said, "you were shot?"

I replied, "yes and stabbed three times, and in a gang at the same age as you are now. If it weren't for my high-school guidance counselor and God allowing me divine retribution, I wouldn't be here right now. I'd be dead or in a jail cell."

I proceeded with suturing as I was halfway through an impeccable job and asked, "Little brother have you ever heard of Malcolm X?"

He replied, "We learned about him in school, he was a political activist back in the sixties that changed his life around and was assassinated by a plot designed by J Edgar. Hoover and the FBI."

I was proud and said, "Wow, look at you, you were taught that and retained the information from school, you're pretty smart huh? And all this time you have your mama thinking you're the reincarnation of the rapper Eazy-E from NWA." We both began to laugh as the tension eased and we spoke cordially like two brothers on a street corner. You wouldn't have thought we were in an emergency room anymore with the joviality that took over the room.

As we spoke candidly, I was able to finish up without him feeling any pain and telling him about my life story. The more I spoke the more intrigued he became by me. I eventually wrapped up the procedure and although he had stitches all over his face he was pleased with my meticulousness and so was I.

I said, "young man, wait here, and went to my locker to grab a copy of my Malcom X autobiography and pleaded with him to read it. He promised me that he would, and I spoke to his grandmother and said I would do my best to remain in this young man's life as a mentor, a brother, a friend, or just a confidante if he ever needed me or she felt over-whelmed and saw any slither of him backsliding in the wrong direction.

I further prescribed antibiotics, pain medication and instructed her to bring him back to the emergency room in 5-7 days for suture removal. I told her to watch for signs of infection; too hot to touch, redness or swelling around the suture sight, fever, increased pain or tenderness around the wound, pus or blood leaking from the sutures, which may have a foul odor, and swollen lymph nodes.

She replied, "wow, that's a lot of information to assimilate at my old age."

I stated, "Ma'am I know it is, so I'll tell you what I'll do to ease that burden. What I'm going to do goes against hospital policy but I will give you my personal cell phone number so you can call me directly at any time of the day or night if you sense anything is wrong, and I'll even go as far as to come to your house and treat him myself if you can't bring him in; Again Ma'am, although this goes against hospital policy, If I can do anything in my power to save your grandson's life then I will do it without any hesitation. If I can save just one person's life, I'd feel like my humanistic goal to society is fulfilled.

She smiled and replied, "thank you, young man, we need more Doctor's like you on this earth to help take care of our people, it really makes a big difference in how we receive quality healthcare."

I stated, "I'm a PA-Student doing my ER residency ma'am."

She replied, "Same difference and I will have you treat me or anyone that I know over a doctor here any day. The doctors at this hospital come into your room and are in and out, in under 5 minutes. They don't even look you in the eye when they speak to you and treat you as if you're just another number on their list of people to see for the day." I assured her that was unfortunate and that I was different. God and the universe insist we meet in this lifetime, here and now for a purpose, which is to help. I further explained that I was a man of my word and reiterated that I would do my best to assist in any way possible.

Throughout the next week, I made it my prerogative to stay in touch with this young man and asked his grandmother how his convalescent was going over the course of the next few days? She stated that "he was doing well and took everything I said seriously. He began to stray away from his gang of "bloods" and even read the autobiography of the Malcolm X book that I gave to him."

He came in the next week for suture removal, and I was enthusiastic and proud of how minimal the scars were. They were so thin that you could barely see them unless you stared at them intently.

While removing the sutures, the young man stated, "By the way I read the entire Malcolm X book and I want to change my life, the way that he did, I want to be a doctor."

I told him "That was phenomenal to hear but applying yourself to Medical school is a huge task that takes a lot of self-determination and will power."

He replied, "after everything I've been through if I can channel all the energy, that I put forth into being down for my gang, I know I can complete medical school."

I replied, "Well, get on that path, and if you fall off the path, dust yourself off, get up, and get back on that path again, develop alligator skin and be tough as nails, I know that you can do this. I have all the faith in the world in you that you can make it. I'll make sure to do everything in my power to help see you through to my end. Finish high-school and get as many A's as you possibly can, because from here on out everything that you do matters. You make sure to have a plan and stick to it. If you fail to plan, then plan to fail. Be sure to never take the word *"no"* for an answer, listen to your teachers and above all else stay away from naysayers, they will distract you and divert you from your plan, which will only reduce your energy and shake up your confidence. Be bold and be proud to be black. Use your brain and make prudent decisions. This won't be easy, but it will be fun, challenging but fun. Exercise and stay in shape. A sharp body behooves a sharp mind. And if there is ever anything that you need, do not hesitate to call me."

He replied, "Thank you for everything you did for me Sir. You have changed my life in every way, and I will not let you down, you have my word." I said, "You've already made me proud by taking the first step to a new life and you can never let me down." With that being said, we parted ways. I hugged his grandmother and told her, "Thank you for allowing me the opportunity to treat your grandchild, I have no doubt in

Aim High Push Hard

my mind that he will be just fine.

Chapter 13

Residency#3

I embarked on my new journey, *Primary care. Primary care* is the day-to-day healthcare given by a health care provider to a patient in the community. Typically, this provider acts as the first point of contact, as the main point of continuing care for patients within a healthcare system and coordinates other specialist care that the patient may need through referrals. Patients commonly receive primary care from professionals such as a primary care physician, a physician assistant or a nurse practitioner. Contingent upon the nature of the health condition, patients may then be referred for secondary or tertiary care. My team consisted of medical assistants and other support team members.

Whom, I was to consistently communicate with about medical needs and progress of all the patients on the days docket.

My primary care clinic location was a ten-minute drive away from where I grew up, but I was over that part of my life at this point and promised myself not to even drive past my old neighborhood to get to my residency clinic. I didn't want any distractions at all. I had complete *mindfulness*, which was the ability to remain focused in a world full of distractions.

My preceptor, who was also the owner of the clinic, was Dr. Afre. He was from Ethiopia, Addis Ababa to be specific. He was humble as a slice of humble pie, hard-working and diligent with his patients, who were all mostly Ethiopian. He arrived to the clinic promptly at 8:30am and see patients until 12:30pm. We would have lunch, which consisted of Injera, which is a sour flatbread used in Ethiopian and Eritrean cuisine that is thicker than a crepe but thinner than a pancake and has a delightfully sour taste. *We ate the injera with Doro Wat (Ethiopian-style spiced chicken stew), Mula-Asa (Ethiopian Pan-Fried Fish) spiced red-*

lentils, Quick Gomen (Ethiopian Spiced Greens). We washed this heart-healthy meal down with green tea. We did this every day of the week during our lunch period; it was a ritual that I took great pride in.

Albeit, I was from West-Africa, I felt gratification in knowing that in East-Africa they ceased everything they were doing to eat lunch together despite how rigorous their day was. That told me they were an easy-going culture of people who were unified and believed in profound cultural values. Not only did they believe these values to be as true today as they were in Ethiopia's primitive years, but they also practiced them daily, and I truly believe, there is something genuine to be said about that.

At 1:00pm we would get back to treating patients until 3:00pm. Subsequently, Dr. Afre would drive forty-five minutes to an hour to Baltimore city, and work at the Baltimore city men's detention center from 3pm-11pm. This man was imposing to me! The fact that he was three times my age and could sustain the physical stamina and mental fortitude to work from 8:30am to 11:00pm daily instilled in me a stellar work ethic that I thought I had, but obviously I hadn't, because I wasn't accustomed to working so many hours in one day. Then driving to Baltimore and back to D.C. every day was another adventure within itself. I felt like I had it easy up until meeting this diligent working Physician.

I later ascertained from Dr. Afre that the reason he worked an additional job was so that he could use the monetary funds to allocate to his primary care clinic because it wasn't making enough money quarterly to sustain his clinic and keep it thriving. He had to pay $63,000 to keep his primary care clinic afloat yearly. This was astonishing to me. That his clinic and patients meant that much to him, that he would work extra hours to keep it open by any means necessary.

The following day I was punctual at 8:30am precisely, bright-eyed, bushy tailed and ready for the day's duties. A typical day for me consisted of overviewing the morning requisition sheet for all the patients for that day and combing through their medical history for any inadequacies that may not have been caught earlier and to bring them to

Dr. Afre's attention before each patient arrived to the clinic. By doing things this way I assured myself to stay ahead of the day's formidable obstacles that may impose a stumbling-block.

Dr. Afre took note of my enthusiasm and proactive nature and gave me a small pat on the back, added by an atta-boy, which made me feel jubilant and proud of the work I accomplished. It was an intrinsic happiness that money could not buy.

I saw patients with ailments ranging from *Hypertension, Diabetes-Mellitus (Type I and Type II), Epilepsy, Bronchitis, Emphysema, Asthma, Headaches, Tension Type Migraines, Cluster Headaches, Fibromyalgia, Bladder infections. Sexually transmitted Infections such as Chlamydia, Gonorrhea, Herpes Virus Tye I and Type II, Pelvic Inflammatory Infections, Urinary Tract Infections, Fever of Unknown Origin. Nosebleeds, Attention Deficit Hyperactive Disorder, Attention Deficit Disorder, Minor Burns, Rashes, Menopause Screenings, Benign Prostatic Hypertrophy, Sprains, Broken Bones, Swelling In The Arms or Legs. To Low Testosterone, Pernicious Anemia, and Iron Deficiency.*

Aim High Push Hard

Any and everything that was on that requisition sheet, I assisted Dr. Afre in working up. I treated patients until he felt comfortable enough to let me off the leash and treat patients on my own. Which only took a week. By week two Dr. Afre ruminated over ten percent of the notes from patients I treated on my own and asked me questions about why I chose the test I chose? If I could have chosen a cheaper diagnostic test? *(X-Ray Vs. CT-Scan)* or a cheaper medication? *(Avelox Vs. Ciprofloxacin)* as these patients were from the destitute community surrounding the area and many of them did not have the monetary assets to pay for high costing medications. The last thing I wanted was a patient calling me from the pharmacy stating they could not receive a medication I prescribed because it cost too much.

I understood that he trusted my judgement and it made me push myself to work meticulously, just as he did. I was also able to work faster as the patient volume increased in the clinic from 15 to 25 patients a day. Although, I did not sacrifice speed for accuracy, I learned patients' first and last names. If they had a dog, I recollected the dog's name and asked

Aim High Push Hard

"How is your dog "spade" doing today? I treated every patient as a human being, just how I would want a medical practitioner to treat me.

I submerged myself in the culture of the East African Country, Addis Ababa. Learned intimately what it meant to come from their land. I began reading books written by "His Imperial Emperor Haile Selassie" who was the emperor of Ethiopia from 1930 to 1974. In fact, it was his initiative and ideology which led Ethiopia to become a charter member of the United Nations. As a student Haile Sellasie's most striking attributes was his keen observation. He was said to notice details often ignored by others, which had me in awe. He instilled the importance of education in me, particularly science. Truth has it the people of Ethiopia are regarded in Africa in its entirety as a sovereign nation, this resonated with me as I was proud of the continent that my ancestors hailed from. Today *"His Imperial Majesty Haile Selassie"* is still considered by the Rastafarian's, a spiritual leader- *a divine figure.*

During my third week of Primary Care Residency, while eating Injera, over spicy lentils and Pan-fried fish. I told Dr. Afre about the time when I was twelve years old, and my mom told me to get dressed, that we were going to Disney world, and I was ecstatic but as we began landing, I looked out the window and noticed clay filled roads with Giraffe's, Lions, Zebras and Tigers. Then proceeded to turn to her and say, questionably, "This doesn't look like Disney World" and she responds, "it's Disney World indeed, the African version." He broke out into jovial laughter and thought the story was hilarious. He told everyone in the clinic about it. However, I did not find the story as humorous or fascinating as he did. But it did make me chuckle a bit.

Closing in on my fourth and final week, I increased my pace of seeing patients and working them up. There was a resound around the clinic by my medical team members about my sedulous work-ethic that I performed in the past 4 weeks, as well as my Disney world story as a child.

Dr. Afre had a talk with me over lunch, where he discussed the opportunity and privilege of me coming back to work there after I passed my board exams. I was surprised that he thought so highly of me to offer me a job. I ruminated over the thought of coming back to work there and held it in the utmost regard. I contemplated it feverishly. However, Emergency Medicine abducted my heart. Henceforth, I told him that I would consider it and I was strictly focused on passing my board exams for the time being. I understood that without passing my boards first and foremost, I wouldn't be working at anyone's clinic, urgent care, emergency room, nothing. I would be a Physician Assistant that completed his residency but not able to practice. With that said, we shook hands, exchanged numbers and parted ways. I thanked him vehemently for instilling in me a strong work ethic and the ability and wherewithal to put my patients above all else as the number one priority.

I went home that night and began studying for my board exams, which were in 3 months. I wanted to give myself ample time to study, as well as a birthday gift, so I elected to take my board exam on February 12, 2010. Failure was not an option; I was confident in my abilities to pass my Physician Assistant National Certification Exam and not to belabor the point, but my will to pass this exam exceeded my will to breathe in oxygen. That's how bad I needed to pass this exam.

I opened each book from Physician Assistant school the previous two years and took it from the top. I studied for each test and went over all the notes. The next day I woke up and drove straight to Barnes and Nobles and bought every book on the Physician Assistant National Certification Exam. I even bought flashcards for added measure. I didn't want to take any KAPLAN classes, although I heard they were great at helping prepare you for your board exams.

Again, if you fail to plan then plan to fail! My plan was to sequester myself in the library for twelve to fourteen hours a day and study voraciously until my eyes bled, wipe the blood off with a paper towel and study some more. That is how hungry I was. Compounded with the determination that nothing would distract me from passing this board exam with excellence. That is the discipline that it takes; you may be unable to teach an individual talent. However, you can teach an individual discipline, not just in childhood but in adulthood as well.

Chapter 14

Graduation

The night before graduation my classmates and I drove to Ocean City, Maryland and had a great time dancing the night away in the club. We danced, twirled, twisted and shimmied our little tootsies all over the dance floor. We finally made it to the end of the PA program, and we were all proud. We conversed with one another about our residencies and exchanged dialogue on where we worked and what we did. It was insightful to hear the other students' stories and to see how different theirs were from mine. Some had a difficult time with their preceptors. Others had dilemmas in finding a suitable hospital or clinic that would take students.

My incoming class of 2007 began with thirty-four students, in the end, only eleven students graduated. It was the first year the University of Maryland Eastern Shore took on so many students. I'm happy they did take us all on because I was among the last two students out of the thirty-four to be granted acceptance. I graduated at the top 1% percentile of my class. Out of the thirty-four students, only two of us matriculated from other schools. This was no small task. Many students had deaths in their family, work, children and other prioritizing things that kept them from being at school full-time. Albeit some of the students who graduated with me also had those similar extraordinary issues. The age range of our graduates was 23 years/old to upwards of 50/years old. So never let anyone tell you that you are too old or too young to go after your dreams. What God has meant for you is for you, and all that you must do is walk that path. Be an annihilator of fear and the rest will happen naturally. If it is God's will, so let it be.

The next day was graduation, on December 12, 2009. For some reason, all throughout my educational years, graduation ceremony always felt like a church revival to me, and given that it spans *three hours, it's nearly as long.* My eyes began brimming with tears.

Ruminating on the long, sleepless nights, and grueling days of going to school percolating through my brain A brother made it, can you believe it? Against all odds, a brother made it out!

I was incredulous that I was actually graduating. I knew that I would, but I just could not believe it. I had flashbacks of my life and where I came from. I kept asking myself, "How many people who came from the ills of the ghetto made it this far? and Achieved this prestigious accomplishment?" All my childhood friends that were murdered, the rest that were arrested; the ones who were strung out on drugs or had countless babies in high school. I did this for them. I did this for every little boy and girl growing up in the urban areas of America with a dream.

When the graduation commencement announcer called my name to walk across the stage and accept my degree, my knees buckled, my sugar dropped, my heart into atrial flutter as I leaped out of the chair and looked up into the sky and whispered, "Thank you God, I couldn't have done this without you." My mother and younger brother were there hooting and hollering. It was an exhilarating feeling that's ineffable to explain. Anyone who's had the honor and pleasure of passing a post-baccalaureate program in medicine knows exactly what I mean. I strutted my way across the stage and shook the commencement announcer's hand as I said, "Thank you sir, this is the greatest accomplishment of my life."

Chapter 15

Board Exams

February 12, 2010; *my twenty-seventh birthday, what a day to take an exam.* You know my mantra? **"GO Hard or GO Home—Leave all the chips on the table baby, let them fall where they may."** The time to take the PANCE had finally arrived! This was the culmination of all the blood, sweat, and tears I poured into this program. It was an arduous road but nothing that lasts in this life comes easy. As the old saying goes *"No Pain-No Gain."*

It was time to get rid of the filters. Make my life my favorite movie. Live my favorite character. Write my own scripts. Direct my own story. Be my biography. Make my own documentary, on me. Nonfiction. Live, not recorded. **Time to aim high, push hard and catch that hero I've**

been chasing*, see if the sun will melt the wax that holds my wings or if the heat is just a mirage. Live my legacy now.*

It was a scary proposition to sit for the board exams. The PANCE exam consists of five 60-minute sections. Yes, you read that right, it is a 5-hour exam! Each section has 60 questions, giving you 1 minute to complete each question. A total of 45 minutes of break time is allotted to you. You are responsible for managing this time. If you leave the exam room during a 60-minute section, this time will be taken away from your actual exam time. You will also not be able to access your locker or materials. Conversely, you could go check your locker during your allotted break period as long as you stayed under that 45-minute threshold. I didn't plan on taking any breaks or checking my locker. The exam cost was $550, that isn't refunded if you fail the board exam. I think that should be repealed.

There is nothing allowed in the test room: no gum, no water, no candy, no napkins to blow your nose if you sneeze, you get the idea. A digital fingerprint will be utilized upon entering and leaving out of the exam room. There will be paper, pencil, and earplugs provided to you.

Furthermore, it takes anywhere from four days to two weeks to receive your test scores. That tedious process should be repealed as well. Why should it take a month to receive scores on a multiple-choice exam? What's the point of artificial intelligence if you're still going to have to wait four weeks to receive test scores that can be calculated within 10 seconds on a computer? It's not like you must write out your answers. They are either wrong or right after you finish taking the test. One plus one equals two. Two plus two equals four, last time I checked, correct? Simple logic, you would think? But hey (Go Figure!). It's not as if someone is in the back grading the test scores manually. I feel like the trepidation the test taker must endure until he or she ascertains their board exam results is futile. I'm not lamenting, that is just my two cents.

I studied voraciously the previous three months. I did what I needed, I lived to learn. My plan was to Follow my intuition, and not to second guess myself on any of the questions. Read the question in its entirety, then gaze over the multiple-choice questions, which some were "K" type questions, meaning, (there was more than one possible answer per question, these questions are tricky, but I persevered). Go back to the question and pull the trigger, all under 60 seconds. Some questions were easier than others, so I answered those in 20-30 seconds, which left me plenty of time remaining to answer the difficult questions.

I had a good night's rest the night prior and woke up to drink an orange juice and scarf down a granola bar. I didn't want to consume much water in order to decrease the need to go to the restroom frequently, which would cut into my exam time. I did not want to check my locker because I projected enough self-awareness to know that I would begin going over questions that I already completed in my head and be ambivalent about my answers, which would decrease my confidence and perhaps dissuade me from answering the next block of sixty questions to the best of my ability.

I had a pristine focus like a prism, and I was on a mission. I completed the exam in four and a half hours and walked out confidently.

Aim High Push Hard

Went across the street to Woodmont Grill in Bethesda, Maryland. Ordered myself a Hawaiian Ribeye Steak-Medium Rare, Bake Potato with all the trimmings and a glass of Chardonnay. Not the Kendall Jackson they sell at the liquor store. I was so enamored with the way I pursued that exam that I knew glory was upon me. I asked the waiter "to bring me the best Chardonnay you have in your wine cellar." I felt like George Jefferson from the sit-com "The Jefferson's" I was moving on up to the east side, to a deluxe apartment in the sky.

Within the next two to four weeks, I received my exam results and I passed with flying colors. I am now a Board-Certified Physician Assistant. Now that's the definition of Aiming High and Pushing Hard.

Chapter 16

Conclusion

I wrote this book so I could have a written record to hold myself accountable to. I wrote this book so you can hold me to task and remind me of what I forgot. I circled back to prior times: lessons learned, repeated and revisited. I noticed that the realizations arrived quickly, the learning took time, **and the livin' was the hardest part.**

My first twenty years were where I learned the value of values. Through discipline and deep affection, I learned respect, accountability, creativity, courage, perseverance, fairness, service, good humor, and a spirit of adventure in ways that some people might consider abusive, but I remember as tough love, and I wouldn't give back one ass whupping for the value of the values that my mother impressed upon me. I thank her for that.

When I began writing this book two years ago, in 2021, my life, like yours, was intercepted by a catastrophic air-borne communicable disease called COVID-19. A pandemic, which morphed into several different *detrimental* and more widespread COVID-19 variants—such as Alpha, Delta, Gamma and Omicron—all became more contagious mostly due to changes in their spike proteins. Spike proteins determine a virus' ability to attach onto and replicate within human cells, thus making it more volatile. Omicron is now the predominant strain in the United States, in part because it can surpass immunity offered by vaccines and boosters.

Which is why The Centers For Disease Control recommends citizens of the United States of America to receive yearly vaccine booster injections. Variants, like Delta and Omicron; Its disruption in our lives became ***inevitable.*** We had to stay at home, social distance, and wear masks for protection. We couldn't go to work, we lost jobs, and loved ones, and we never truly knew when it would end. We were scared, we were angry. Each of us had to make sacrifices, pivot, deal, and persist— we had to get relative. Sometimes you don't realize how strong you are until being strong is the only choice you have.

Then drama introduced itself in the name of the George Floyd murder. I saw him on the ground screaming in agony for help and calling out for his mother. That brute, Derek Chauvin's knee firmly placed on George Floyd's neck at the carotid-artery bifurcation for twelve long minutes, while other officers stood by doing absolutely nothing; I felt an instant shock of vicariousness through George Floyd's helpless eyes overcome me. As he gasped for air, I was in a trance of the many times Police Officer's had their knees on my neck as I gasped for what felt like my final breath. Mentally it haunts me, I try to repress it and move on with my life.

The Murder by Derek Chauvin against George Floyd and Its disruption in our lives soon became **inevitable** as well. There were protests, riots, looting, fear and outrage. The unjust murder sparked a social justice revolution in America and around the world, and as racism reared its ugly head into the spotlight once again, we were reminded that *ALL Lives* couldn't matter until *Black Lives Matter* more.

COVID-19 and the murder of George Floyd, forced us inward, literally quarantined us to search our souls for a better way forward. In doing so we took inventory of our lives; and who we are in them—what we care about, what matters, what our priorities are. We got to know our families, children and ourselves better. We cried, we prayed, we read, we wrote, we listened, we screamed, we spoke out, we marched, we helped others in need. But how much did we change ***for good—it's sake and forever?*** Months after George Floyd, there was Breonna Taylor, a 26-year-old African American woman, who was fatally shot in her Louisville, Kentucky apartment on March 13, 2020, when seven police officers forced entry into her apartment. She was an Emergency Medical Technician, who was murdered while sleeping in her bed.

For those of us who survived similar traumatic experiences in our lives, when and how we see the benefits of what we went through during those turbulent times is relative. All that we can do is to work individually to make the justified changes for a more value driven and righteous tomorrow.

The other reason I wrote this book was so it can be a useful tool and serve as a lending hand if you need it, that it might teach you something, inspire you, make you laugh, remind you, help you forget, and arm you with some life tools to better march forward as more of yourself. As for me? ***I haven't made all A's in the art of livin' but I do give a damn, and I'll take an experienced "C" over an ignorant "A" any day.***

I always believed that the science of satisfaction is about learning when, and how, to get a handle on the formidable challenges we face in life. When you can design your own weather,

blow in the breeze, control your own destiny and shape your own life. When you're stuck in the storm, pray for luck and make the best of it. We all have scars, we'll get more, they ultimately build character and mold us into who we become. **So rather than struggle against time and waist it, let's dance with time and redeem it, because we don't live longer when we try not to die, we live longer when we're too busy livin'.**

As I've navigated the weather in my own life, getting relative with the inevitable has been a key to my success. **Relatively,** we are livin'. Life is our resume. It is our story to tell, and the choices we make write the chapters. Can we live in a way where we look forward to looking back? **Inevitably,** we are going to die. Our eulogy, our story, will be told by others and forever introduce us when we are gone.

The Soul Objective. Begin with the end in mind.

What's your story? This is mine so far.

Aim High Push Hard, **Just keep Livin'**

GOD BLESS, I LOVE YOU ALL UNCONDITINALLY!

~ GodSpeed

www.ingramcontent.com/pod-product-compliance
Lightning Source LLC
Chambersburg PA
CBHW040455240426
43663CB00033B/3